An Unfi·
Mother

D1589505

WITHDRAWN
992683824 3

To
My family - Jem and Emma

An ~~Un~~fit Mother

How to get your Health,
Shape and Sanity back
after childbirth

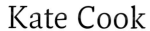

Kate Cook

with Lucy Wyndham-Read

Collins

First published in 2008 by Collins, an imprint of HarperCollins Publishers Ltd.
77-85 Fulham Palace Road
London W6 8JB

www.collins.co.uk
Collins is a registered trademark of HarperCollins Publishers Ltd.

Text © Kate Cook 2008
Illustrations © HarperCollins Publishers 2008

Illustrations by Alice Tait. The illustrator would like to thank George Wu, Vanessa James and Scott Chambers for all of their help.

6 5 4 3 2 1
11 10 09 08

The author asserts her moral right to be identified as the author of this work. All rights reserved. No parts of this publication may be reproduced, stored in a retrieval system or transmitted, in any form or by any means, electronic, mechanical, photocopying, recording or otherwise, without the prior permission of the publishers.

A catalogue record for this book is available from the British Library.

ISBN 978-0-00-725974-8

Collins uses papers that are natural, renewable and recyclable products made from wood grown in sustainable forests. The manufacturing processes conform to the environmental regulations of the country of origin.

This is a general reference book and although care has been taken to ensure the information is as up-to-date and accurate as possible, it is no substitute for professional advice based on your personal circumstances. Consult your doctor before making any major changes to your diet.

Colour Origination by Colourscan, Singapore
Printed in Singapore by Imago

The author would like to thank:
Jenny Irving, Melissa McCrae (Aveda), David Samson, Kim Upton, Lisa Neubronner, Catriona Muir, Camilla Schneiderman (Divertimenti), Naava Carma, Seki Tejani, Jill Prodenchuk and in particular, my wonderful team at The Nutrition Coach – Sanna Anderson and Kim Porter.

Gloucestershire County Council	
LS*	
992683824 3	
Askews	15-Jan-2009
613.704	£9.99

Contents

Introduction

If you are flicking through this in the bookshop, trying to focus through bleary, non-seeing eyes and feeling like you drank 20 glasses of wine last night, either you have the hangover from hell or you are a new mother. Welcome to the tribe, Sister.

That jolly teacher at the pre-natal class didn't really tell you about the afterwards, did she? Preparation, preparation, preparation is all very well but an ounce of theory is worth a tonne of practice – how did you really know what it was actually going to be like? Having a baby seemed like an unreal dream right from the telling your parents bit through to the excitement of shopping for the baby's room. And the actual birth. Well, it all seemed so sort of remote and kind of easy in theory. Just push something the size of a melon through tiny little hole. Easy.

After all the attention of the actual event and day, and the visits and all the presents, and after all the flowers have died and all the balloons have gone limp, what are you left with? A little bundle of joy, sure – but no instructions of how to operate and boy, do you now know the meaning of tired. The tired that says, 'So what if all the washing up hasn't been done for a week?', and you can't be bothered to find some clothes, any clothes, let alone matching socks. Instead, you have resorted to going *out* of the house in your huge grey, elephant-like unsexy sweat pants. 'Blimey,' you say, to no one in particular, 'I am really losing it big time.' Actually, you might be saying it to yourself and just moving your lips.

Once the really treacle tired bit has passed – and it will, although it may not seem like it just now – it does get easier (proper promise; the night feeding does stop). Then it is about time to start to at least think about reclaiming not only your old body, but also your mind, sanity and the, well, the *you* part of you.

It feels like that naughty stork dumped the baby and then made off with your old jeans and dumped a much smaller pair that you seem unable to get into. Frankly, this is beginning to depress you. Not only has the stork stolen your jeans but he took away your old life, too. 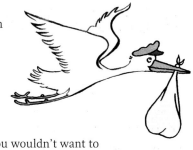 Now don't get me wrong, you wouldn't want to go back entirely to the old you, but it would be nice to have something of that old dynamic, non-mummsy self back – the one without the trail of tot-snot down the front.

So who's actually writing this book?

Fear not – Lucy Wyndham-Read (on exercise) and I, Kate Cook, are the ones applying for the job of getting you to a really fab place with not only your fitness but your nutrition and the whole of your life and thinking! Well, we like to aim high.

I am a nutritional therapist and life coach with bags of experience. I have seen over 4,500 patients face to face, who I hope I have all helped, at least in some way – and hopefully I am about to help you, too. I believe in seeing nutrition and life in general as something that has to be do-able – and it has to be something that fits in with your lifestyle and the fact that you are human. There is the absolutely perfect way of doing all this and then there is the real way, which you are going to apply to all the information in this wonderful, wonderful book. You are not going to do all of it! So don't feel bad – just try to do some of it. We are not looking for total perfection. You only have to do a bit better than you are now – that's all.

Lucy is the exercise expert and is fitness trainer to the Stars, but is really down to earth and specialises in the no-workout workout – stuff you can do at home and on the hoof rather than having to do exercises in a gym.

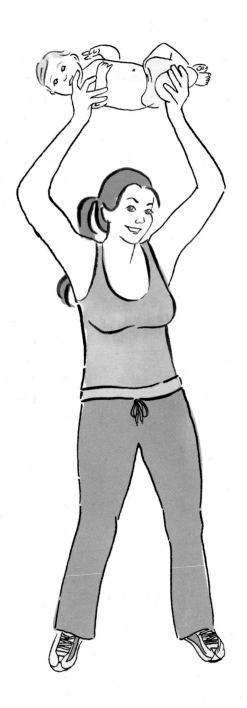

The preparation bit

If you want, you can start to think about your life, nutrition and fitness as soon as you are being wheeled out of the delivery suite. Indeed, the preparation programme is designed for you to start at any time. I introduce you to some good eating habits and Lucy has written some nice 'n easy exercises to get you going. Don't be tempted to start too soon or your stomach muscles may not be knitted together properly – that will make more sense later and Lucy will tell you about that, too – so check it out before you launch into a thousand press-ups.

The nutrition bit

Change happens over a period of time and if you try to change everything all at once, you might keep it up for a week, but then you will certainly think, 'Sod it!' at some point and all the old habits will come roaring back with a vengeance. Think back to how you were at school and how you are now, and of course you have changed and developed, but you haven't had to really make an effort to change. It has just happened organically as you have learnt new strategies that make life easier.

Nutrition is depicted nowadays on the TV as some kind of really strict, joyless discipline. Horrible. Nutrition should be something that is nurturing and flexible. The 'I-am-going-to confiscate-everything-you-ever-liked' image is not helped by the new fad for the reality show where being really nice to people and being really realistic doesn't make good TV – the directors want to give you the impression that nutrition is all or nothing. Whacking people with carrots and humiliating the overweight makes everyone squirm and tune in next week, but does it work for ordinary folk? I get truly intimidated plus I hate people being horrible to each other.

The ultra-militant approach to nutrition gives you the fish and not the fishing rod. While your dominatrix is standing there ready to smack you in the face with the wet kipper you can keep it up (with knees knocking), but once she is gone, you sigh a huge breath of relief and are left wondering what to do next. You are locked into a 'system' and feel disempowered.

This book, then, is about freeing you from the plague of actually dieting for the rest of your life and not just now, but forever. By their very nature, diets mean that you start a diet and then you end a diet, and what do you do when you end the diet? You go back to your old ways and just pile back on the pounds like you always do. I know this because before I was a nutritional therapist, I was trapped into yo-yo dieting and was quite a chunky chipmunk. I looked more like a hamster, actually – a hamster with a fringe. After I learned how to eat I have never, ever dieted ever again. And by the way, I am still a size 10 and not my old size, in case you think I have just stopped caring. Liberation!

So, you just need to know how to eat – and eat this way for life. Full stop. In the food chapter – cunningly called the nutrition bit – I tell you the basics of nutrition so that you know what you are doing

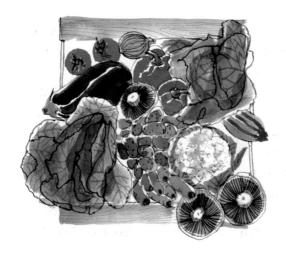

on the eating front. Then, in the next chapter – the
exercise and putting it all together bit! (see
below) – we put all the nutrition info
together with Lucy's exercise stuff so
that you have a very practical, 'What the
Hell am I meant to be doing?' section to
work through.

In the nutrition chapter, I have deliberately not gone
into long descriptions about how your insulin levels
function and how you store glycogen or how cortisol
works in relation to your blood sugar – you can get this
ad nauseum from other tomes. Nor have I been prescriptive about
what you should have to eat every day. Instead, I have made
suggestions for you to adapt to what you do like – you have to
learn how to be flexible and apply what I am telling you right from
the beginning or you will be forever wanting to look over your
shoulder to ask me if a certain food is OK or not. You are almost
certainly over 21 and vaccinated and I trust you to be able to make
up your own mind.

The exercise and putting it all together bit

In this part of the Wonder Tome, Lucy has given you a huge amount
of choice and flexibility in the exercises but, again, they are not
meant to be done to perfection although, of course, if one of the
exercises inspires you to do something, then that is fab – our job
here is done. The only thing Lucy wants you to do for sure, as much
for your sanity as anything else, is to get out there walking on your
pram walks – but all that will become clear later. For the keenies
who follow all the programme and get fabulous results (including
toned butts), that is fine too.

But this chapter is so much more than just a set of exercises.
Together, Lucy and I have created a week-by-week breakdown for

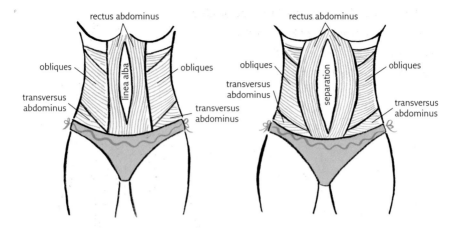

rectus abdominus

rectus abdominus

obliques

obliques

obliques

obliques

linea alba

separation

transversus abdominus

transversus abdominus

transversus abdominus

transversus abdominus

transversus abdominus

transversus abdominus

You need to use all these muscles groups to help get your stomach toned again after the separation that can occur during pregnancy.

the first month, explaining how to combine all your new-found knowledge on food, exercise and being kind to yourself.

The first week is quite detailed – you should get the hang of it with that – then weeks two, three and four are a little more free-flow. You *really* will have got the hang of it by then. By month two you will be cruising and to maintain it is easier than you would have thought.

Look out for Lucy's trainers icon throughout the book when she dispenses sage advice. The owl icon appears when I have something wise to say and helps you differentiate between our voices.

The lifestyle bit

A vital part of getting the *you* back is to rediscover your self-confidence by being nice to yourself and also realising that people are having the same experiences as you. Some of you will find some parts of being a mum easy and other parts hard, and some of you will find the whole thing hard – it depends on you and your personality and on your little one, too. There are babies that pop out good as gold and others, well, they are a bit more of a challenge.

Who knows why that happens? Even one brother can be a little lamb and the other a pickle (polite term). Of course you love them (sometimes not all of the time, but most of the time), but often it is hard not to think of motherhood as an unpaid servant's role – changing nappies, preparing food (if weaning), being woken up in the night and picking up tiny socks. And then there's the realisation of responsibility and in this huge new role it is all too easy to lose yourself and who you are. Of course, you are happy to be Mum, but it would be nice to take the badge off and put your feet up at the local day spa and feel, well, human.

So be nice to yourself, don't give yourself a hard time and do some small things to claw back your confidence and your time – and *you*.

Retire to the bathroom to read the next chapter. (Tiny knock on the bathroom door, turning to manic hammering with Barbie head.) 'Mamma? Mamma? MAAAAMA! MAAAAMA! MA! MA!'

The preparation bit

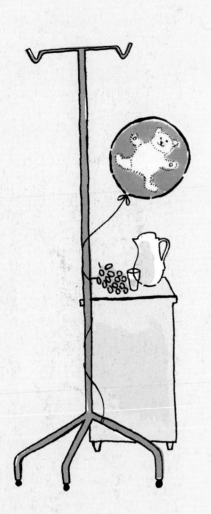
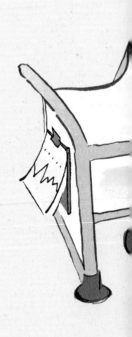

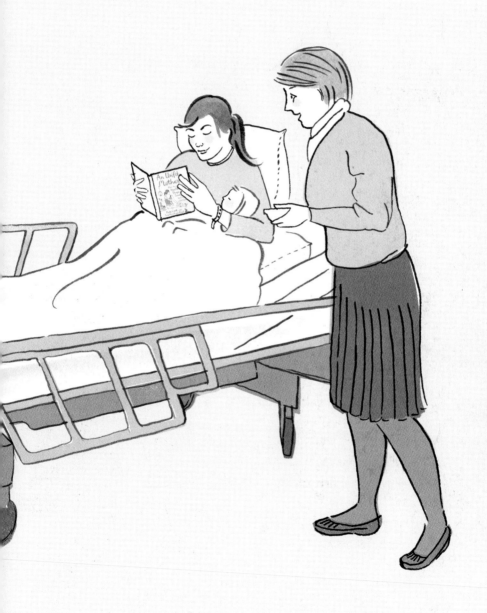

If it's not too late, start NOW

I really hope that you are picking up this book in the bookshop and are having a browse, newly pregnant. I can save you a lot of time and trouble, and I can get you to re-claim those jeans much more quickly – or even a pair of lusciously sexy new ones. All ears? Start now. Yes, you heard right, start now! I am not talking about a slimming diet, goodness no, us nutritional types don't talk in terms of an actual diet, just a better diet, an optimum nutrition diet.

Us Brits have a really poor attitude to food. As I am definitely not a shrink and only a humble nutritionist and wise old owl, I don't really know about all the psychological reasons behind this. However, I do know that lots of parents use food as reward right from a really early age.

* 'Be a good girl and eat up all your food.'
* 'You only get the chocolate chip cookie when you have finished your cabbage.'

Surely, no contest? Gollup down the cabbage and get 'the nice stuff', while holding your nose and practically gagging on the cabbage. You have just been told that cabbage is yucky and that chocolate is nice – a reward, in effect. Years later when we are in charge of our own nutritional destiny as an adult, you can therefore skip straight to the chocolate chip cookies and there is no one there to make you eat that cabbage. 'Oh joy! Tee hee! See if they can *stop* me (etc).'

The downside is that chocolate chip cookies in large amounts cause our girths to expand. And there really is no getting around this. Sorry.

So a great many of us have the concept of reward in food. 'If I am going through a really hard time and I have been good, I need a treat or I will feel deprived.' And if we do have a so-called healthy diet, we bottle up all this goodness and, lo and behold, when the doc tells us that the Stork is due to pay you a visit, you say, '*Great*, now I can eat what I want!' You can't. Sorry.

'Tell us, oh Guru,' I hear you cry, 'Tell us. Oh, what is the secret? What is this Optimum Nutrition Diet that I must follow to be both slim and wise like you, oh great and worthy one?'

The secret is ... that you must:

* Eat loads of fresh and luscious vegetables washed down with pure water.
* Eat plenty of health-giving fruit, some whole grains full of vitamins and minerals.
* Consume fish and a little meat, if you like. That's it!

So remember that:

* A healthy attitude to food saves you an extra trouser size or two.
* Start to look at your nutrition and exercise before you actually get pregnant.
* A splurge from time to time means you are human and not an alien being.

During pregnancy

On my roundup of fresh research victims, my beam of attention turned to my colleague Louise who is now pregnant with number two (a little sibling for the lovely Jasper). Louise is a qualified nutritional therapist who managed to complete her training while Jasper was getting ready to hatch – quite an achievement. So what are her observations about getting back in shape?

Lumps and bumps

Lumps and bumps for a start – bits bulge out where no bits bulged before. That is quite disconcerting, Louise says. When you have been used to being in control of your body, it can be fairly alarming when suddenly, like a magician's balloon at a children's party, your stomach resembles a sausage dog.

The mythical eating for two plot

With Jasper, Louise also feels that she had said a mythical, 'Sod it!' once she found she was pregnant. She let go of her discipline around food. Her portions became massive (definitely 'eating for two'), but as luck would have it, because she was training to be a nutritional therapist, at least her double portions were healthy ones – but too much of a good thing isn't necessarily wonderful. Healthy food is great, healthy food is even great in big portions, but watch the mega giant portions!

This time Louise has wised up to that. Yes, you may feel hungrier; yes, your body is changing and has different needs but it is the quality of the food that is vital, not necessarily the amount. In fact, you only need 200 extra calories in the last three months of your pregnancy. The newly pregnant, 'let's push the "go nuts" button and think about stuffing-the-whole-thing-back-in-the-box of carefulness after a couple of months' attitude is really difficult to overcome once you have had 500 cream buns.

Not impossible, but more difficult. Of course, we all have our moments, but once the moment becomes the whole time – well, who are you trying to kid?

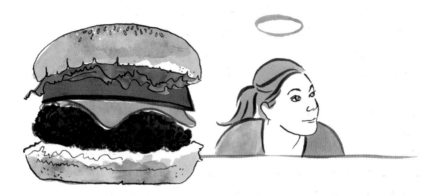

Remembering that you are pregnant and *not* fat is the key. If you are putting on weight, you think, 'Well, who cares anyway?' But this ain't so. Repeat after me, 'I am pregnant and not fat.' In this way, you can really re-educate the way you think about your body – Louise has learnt to really love her pregnant alter ego this time. She feels sexier and more womanly, with curves in all the right places.

Ask any bloke – most men love pregnant women and curvy women; they look, well, they look like women should. Most blokes also hate our obsession with food and being thin. For most men, trying to be thin doesn't even begin to cross the screen of what's important in life, which is why blokes are running the world. They are not using up all that valuable headspace worrying about the size of their butts.

We owe it to our children, therefore, to stop obsessing about our hip and waist measurements and start thinking instead about far more important things – like, for example, how we could do a darned sight better job of running the planet if we were in charge.

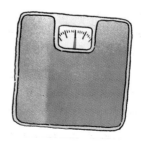

Stop looking at yourself (endlessly!)

Don't spend hours in front of the long mirror in your bedroom, pregnant or not – this is a sure way to get totally paranoid, says Louise. Try to be where you are with your body and not wish your life away dreaming of being thinner or fitter or younger. We spend so much of our time wishing we were something we are not – be where you are now!

Patience

It took Louise much longer than she thought it would to get back her pre-Jasper figure – with a new baby in the house, spending time with her partner and running a house and business, the time to exercise just wasn't there. This time round, though, she is doing more exercise while pregnant, so that she is altogether in better nick.

* Eating a healthier diet throughout pregnancy is key.
* Change your attitude towards your body – you are pregnant and not fat!
* Be patient – you will take time to get back to your pre-pregnancy weight.
* Be kind to yourself.

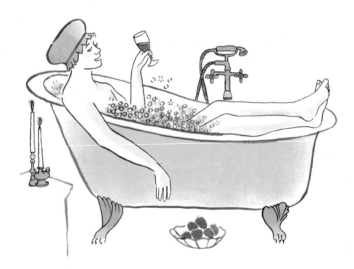

In the hospital

We all know you are not in the hospital for the food. Get someone to bring you some energy-supporting food for when you have had the baby. I know this sounds like being in the movie *Midnight Express*, where you have been transported to some dodgy Turkish jail, and have to rely on the kindness of your family to feed you, but you will thank me later when you get out of there. You could ask for:

* Oatcakes
* Fresh fruit
* Almonds
* Seeds – like pumpkin seeds
* Nut butters
* Bottled water
* Cool bag with hummus, salads, guacamole.

The homecoming
Try to plan ahead and organise one of the following for when you get home. You'll need it.

* Ask someone to fill the fridge with great stuff so that you and the chocolate chip cookie monster stay apart.
* Pay a student/cook to come in and cook simple meals to freeze (or ask your mum).
* Consider a company like www.purepackage.com if you are in London. They will deliver fresh, healthy meals – be sure to tell them you are breastfeeding. (Extra calories needed, honest!)

Start thinking about food

This bit is our gentle stroll into getting your nutritional act together. So relax. Ideally, you would not be reading this when you are desperate to get your body back, you would really have thought about it before giving birth. But let's face it, there's a big difference between the ideal world and reality. Right now, escaping out of the hospital and thinking of eating great healthy food is probably the last thing on your mind. Boring but true. All you need to do for now is get organised.

* Pack your freezer with delicious, nutritious foods – or get someone in (your mum?) to cook some stuff for you. This all sounds like a massive schlep but it will pay *huge* dividends. Freeze enough for a few weeks. Think about:
  - Stews
  - Soups
  - Chicken
  - Fish pies
  - Roasted vegetables
  - Frozen organic veg, such as peas and spinach
* Set up an internet delivery template for your shopping. Can you get your partner to do this?
* Get an organic delivery box stuffed with veggies – great for making simple soups.
* Have a fruit bowl on your kitchen table.
* Snacks – get in hummus and oatcakes together with some nuts and seeds.
* Stock up your cupboards with great stuff (see page 247) and chuck out biscuits and crisps. I am telling you that these will be highly tempting when you are knackered and will be the first thing you reach for – just because they are there.

Think about increasing:

* Veggies and fruit - really obvious!
* Beans and lentils - not everyone's cup of tea, but lentils are easy to cook and you can get pulses like beans and chickpeas from a tin (organic, naturally) - no need for soaking (which involves an element of planning ahead!).
* Eat fresh fish, poultry and lean meats - organic if you can run to it.
* Eat dairy in moderation - just three times a week. You can get calcium and other important minerals from green leafy vegetables and nuts and seeds.

Focus on breakfast

Don't try to do everything 'right', but if you have a proper breakfast you are much more likely to get off to a good start. Breakfast is tempting to skip - don't! Your whole day goes out of whack if you don't get off to a good start. But before I give you some ideas for breakfast, check out your staple ingredients. Make sure you have the following in your home:

* Rice, oat or soya milk or organic bio yoghurt, goat's milk or sheep's milk yoghurt, plain tofu or soya yoghurt.
* Raw, unsalted nuts (almonds, hazelnuts, pecans, Brazils, walnuts, cashews) and/or seeds (sunflower, pumpkin, flaxseeds, hemp, sesame). Keep these in an airtight container in the fridge to protect their essential oils.
* Dried fruit - only as an emergency measure while you wean yourself off sugar; use dried fruit to sweeten porridge if really necessary.

What makes a healthy breakfast?

A good breakfast could be:

* Scrambled eggs on rye toast
* Poached egg with spinach
* Spanish omelette
* Sardines on rye toast with tomatoes
* Porridge made with rolled oats with berries
* Proper muesli with berries and apples (proper meaning not junk food muesli - real muesli is normally found in a health-food shop)
* Other types of bread, like rye and spelt with nut butters, such as cashew nuts
* Yoghurt and berries.

Brilliant breakfasts

The ultimate smoothie

Choose any three of the following fruits:

Apples

Apricots, fresh if in season; if using dried ones, soak them overnight

Bananas

Berries, such as blackberries, blueberries, bilberries, blackcurrants, raspberries, redcurrants, strawberries (fresh or frozen)

Figs, fresh if in season; if using dried ones, soak them overnight

Kiwis

Mangoes

Oranges (if you are not avoiding citrus)

Peaches

Pears

1 Put the fruit with some milk/yoghurt into a blender and add a handful of any nuts or seeds and a handful of oats. Whiz to blend.

2 Vary the amount of liquid depending on the consistency that you prefer, and add an ice cube for a more refreshing blend during the summer. Alter the ingredients for a variation in taste and nutrients.

Muesli

Amaranth

Buckwheat flakes

Barley flakes*

Millet flakes

Oat flakes*

Rice flakes

Rye flakes*

Quinoa flakes

Dried fruit, such as cranberries, raisins, currants, dates, figs, unsweetened flaked coconut, apricots or sultanas

1 Choose any four of the flakes and put 1 tablespoon of each into a bowl. Do not use the items marked with an * if you are following a gluten-free diet.

2 Add 2 tablespoons of any of the dried fruit and also add some nuts and seeds from your storecupboard together with milk or yoghurt.

Variation

In place of the dried fruit, add a grated or chopped apple or pear, or fresh or frozen berries. If using berries, use an 'apple-sized' portion.

Seeded yog-pot

3 tbsp yoghurt

3 tbsp seeds, ground or used whole

Pinch of cinnamon, nutmeg, vanilla essence or ginger

1 Combine all the ingredients in a bowl and enjoy.

2 For variety, substitute 1 tablespoon of nuts for the seeds.

Variation

Add grated or chopped apple or pear, or fresh or frozen berries. If using berries, use an 'apple-sized' portion.

Porridge

2 tbsp jumbo porridge oats (regular oats are fine)

60ml (2fl oz) water

1 tbsp yoghurt or milk, or oat milk or rice milk as alternatives

1 tbsp nuts or seed mix

Pinch of cinnamon, nutmeg, vanilla essence or ginger

1 Mix the oats and water in a pan and bring to the boil. Reduce the heat and leave to simmer for 1 minute. Alternatively, soak the oats the night before, in just enough water to cover them and heat in the morning.

2 Add the yoghurt or milk together with the nuts or seed mix and the spices. Stir together and eat.

Organic free-range eggs on . . .

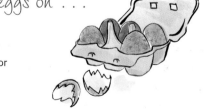

2 organic free-range eggs

Soda bread, rye, spelt or other wheat-free bread, or rice, corn or oatcakes or Ryvita

Spread, such as hummus or pesto

1 Boil the eggs in a small saucepan of water for 4 minutes for a soft yolk, or poach in water for the same length of time.

2 Spread the bread, oatcakes or Ryvita with the hummus or pesto and serve with the freshly-cooked eggs alongside.

Scrambled eggs

2 organic free-range eggs
1 tsp crème fraîche, yoghurt or milk
1/2 tbsp extra virgin olive oil or knob
　of unsalted butter
Soda bread, rye, spelt or other
　wheat-free bread, or rice, corn or
　oatcakes or Ryvita
Spread, such as hummus, pesto
　(very good with eggs), unsalted
　butter or non-hydrogenated
　spread
Freshly ground black pepper,
　turmeric or paprika

Herbs to garnish, such as dill, chives
　or parsley, preferably fresh, if not,
　dried will do

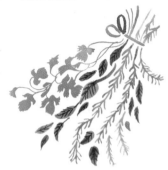

1 In a jug or bowl, beat together the eggs and crème fraîche, yoghurt or milk. Heat the oil or butter in a medium-sized saucepan, but don't allow it to smoke.

2 Add the eggs to the saucepan and cook to the consistency you prefer.

3 Meanwhile, spread the bread with the topping of your choice and serve with the scrambled eggs, garnished with the black pepper, turmeric or paprika and the fresh or dried herbs.

Variation

For those mornings when you fancy something extra with your eggs, grill or steam some tomatoes, or steam any other vegetable. Steaming only takes a few minutes and is a great way to add additional colour and flavour to your plate. Try broccoli, asparagus, spinach, chard, mangetout or any other vegetables you have to hand. Additionally, you can add a few strips of smoked salmon.

Soda bread

25g (1oz) unsalted butter
225g (8oz) non-wheat flour
1/2 tsp baking powder (xantham gum, if you are avoiding gluten)

300ml (1/2 pint) buttermilk – if you are eliminating dairy, use soya
Handful of sunflower or pumpkin seeds

1 Preheat the oven to 200°C (400°F/Gas 6).
2 In a mixing bowl, rub the butter, flour and baking powder together and then add the milk.
3 Knead briefly into a round or oval and bake on a baking sheet in the centre of the oven for 30 minutes until risen and golden.

Off-limit foods!

Let me declare right now, that I really hate the idea of 'off-limit' foods because the very idea makes you want to go out and eat as much as you possibly can, just to prove that they are not actually off-limits at all. Because you are super intelligent (all us girls are!), you will know that if you eat a lot of crappy, junk foods filled with fat, sugar or refined carbohydrates you won't get to your goals because they make you put on weight ... but you don't need me telling you that.

So, here's a really blindingly obvious list of things that you might want to give a miss because: a) they are fattening and b) they are really crappy foods that you wouldn't give to a starving hamster:

* Cream buns
* Crisps
* Biscuits
* Loads of white bread
* Processed meals
* Burgers, pizzas and takeaways in general
* Fizzy drinks
* Cakes
* Loads of butter and fatty spreads and dips.

Some gentle exercising

And now for something a little more energetic, even though we are starting gently. This section is for all you motivated types or completely crazy bods who want to get started while still on the delivery trolley. The exercises in this section are specifically designed so that they are safe straight out of the delivery room – but, of course, being sensible, you might want to check with your GP first.

Lucy has devised some really simple Pilates-type exercises for this section to knit back a few of those dodgy muscles that get roughed around a tad in pregnancy. Together with the nutrition tips, they are a foundation for what is to come later. This section isn't so much a plan as an amble. It's an introduction to sensible stuff about exercise and eating. The meat and potatoes of a kick-ass programme are in the nutrition and exercise bits, which you could start much earlier, should you want to, as long as you have your doc's approval.

 Get someone to go out and get the following kit for you:

* A Swiss ball. If you don't know what this is, well, do you remember the Space Hopper of old? In short, this is a big bouncy ball, only minus the 'ears'. It's a great investment.
* A long piece of string – I am sure you are intrigued as to what you could possibly do with this, but it will get your waist back into shape (not on its own, obviously).
* A pack of coloured sticky notes.
* A mat for floor work or else a low-tech version: a towel

The following exercises – The Super Seven – are designed to work on your deepest muscles. You will be building your strength from the inside, concentrating on your core muscles first. They will draw in your waist muscles, tone up your pelvic floor and you will soon be laughing with confidence (I bet the doctors didn't tell you about the 'squeak and you leak', did they?) – and we *will* get those boobs heading north again.

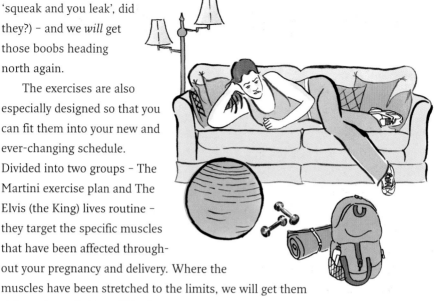

The exercises are also especially designed so that you can fit them into your new and ever-changing schedule. Divided into two groups – The Martini exercise plan and The Elvis (the King) lives routine – they target the specific muscles that have been affected through-out your pregnancy and delivery. Where the muscles have been stretched to the limits, we will get them tight and toned. You will be fit and strong in no time!

The Martini exercise plan

These exercises can be done any time, any place, anywhere. You are too young to remember that ad campaign for Martini, to be sure, but still the point is that you can do these exercises in the line at the bank, in the bus or at the post office – like something out of the *Full Monty* – or while cleaning your teeth, changing your baby's nappy or drinking a cup of tea. I recommend you use your stickers dotted around the house as a constant visual reminder to do them, or you will get to Friday and not even have started.

Metabolic rate

Metabolism is the rate at which your body burns calories and by exercising you can increase the number of calories you burn, naturally increasing your metabolism. So if you are struggling for motivation to do another set of your exercises, just think how many extra calories you will be burning off.

The ice maiden

What it does: This exercise will give you oodles of confidence as you engage with your body's correct posture – your posture is really knocked out of whack in pregnancy as you are compensating all the time because it's like having a huge bag of spuds up your jumper. You have to lean back or you would fall over. Increased weight on the bust, a growing tummy – need I say more? Good posture makes you look lighter, younger and makes your boobs look even bigger. Put one of those sticky notes near the kettle to remind you to do this. If you are feeling artistic, draw a picture of a stick to remind you to keep your back straight.

1 Stand up and imagine that someone has just dropped an ice cube down the back of your shirt.

2 You automatically squeeze your shoulders together and lift your chest up.

3 While you are at it pull in your stomach muscles. Hold for several seconds, release and then repeat as many times as you need to get into the habit of always standing like this.

Squeeze please, Louise

What it does: The benefits are that not only will it help you get a toned and pert rear-of-the-year-type bottom, you will also be increasing your metabolic rate – the more toned your muscles are, the more calories the body burns. This exercise is also very simple – do it while you brush your teeth. Cue sticky piece of paper. Draw a large bottom on it and stick it on your mirror. Keep squeezing girls.

1 Stand up straight. Perfect posture please, making sure that your knees are soft (in other words, not locked out).

2 Squeeze that bum as tightly as you can. Hold. Then slowly release.

3 Repeat 10 times. As you get stronger hold the squeeze for longer.

Belt up

What it does: This exercise engages your deepest tummy muscle – it is a muscle that is like a corset and should keep everything in. Naturally, during pregnancy this muscle will have been over-stretched and now you need to reel it back in. Your lower back is also strengthened with this one. You need this exercise to get back that hourglass gorgeousness. Do this one in the morning while you are preparing breakfast – go on, whack a sticky note on the cooker hood to remind you.

What you will need: That piece of string.

1   Stand up and pull in your tummy muscles really tight.

2   Tie the piece of string around your waist

3   Keep those tummy muscles tight or your stomach will cut into the string. Cruel? You have to suffer to be beautiful.

4   Breathe normally for as long as you can stand it. As each day passes, you'll find you can do this for longer.

The Elvis (the King) lives routine

While The Martini exercise plan can be done wherever you like, the four exercises in this routine need to be done one after the other. But it will only take you a couple of minutes, promise. Aim to do the routine every day and always warm up by first marching for a couple of minutes on the spot.

When's the best time to do them? In your downtime, as little as it is, perhaps in front of the television. Stick a sticker on the screen. That'll annoy your partner.

Elvis the pelvis

What it does: This exercise has amazing benefits. It helps strengthen the deepest abdominal muscles, drawing in your waist as well as building strength in the lower back.

You will need: A mat or towel.

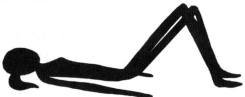

1 Lie on your back on the mat, with your knees bent and feet flat on the floor. Keep your head and shoulders on the floor and put your arms by your sides, with palms facing down.

2 Keep your spine in a neutral position, meaning in line with your hips and shoulders and not arched.

3 Breathe in with a big breath through your nose and then gently exhale through your mouth as you pull your navel towards your spine, tilting your pelvis so the pubic bone lifts and your lower back presses into the floor.

4 Hold for 2 seconds, release and return to the start.

5 Repeat 12 times. Rest and then get on with another 12.

The 'Kegel', don't pee gal

What it does: Imagine that at the bottom of your stomach there is a hammock-shaped muscle that is holding everything up – boy, has it gone a bit saggy after all that's been sitting in it for the last few months. This exercise is therefore designed to help tone up the pelvic floor muscle, or that hammock. Don't do this exercise when you are really having a pee as you could give yourself an infection, but you could do it after you are done – just sit there for 10 seconds longer and give them a squeeze. Try a sticky note on the loo paper holder.

What you need: A mat or towel.

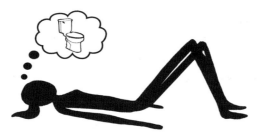

1 First, to identify the muscle, imagine you are sitting on the loo and you want to stop peeing – the one you are squeezing right now is your pelvic floor.

2 Lie face up on the mat with knees bent and feet flat on the floor. Keep your head and shoulders on the floor and put your arms by your sides, with palms facing down. You can also do this exercise while standing up.

3 Squeeze your pelvic floor muscle. Hold for a count of 10 seconds, then release.

4 Do this 12 times. Rest and then get on with another 12.

 As many as one in three women suffer from stress incontinence after childbirth as a result of their hammock swinging low and loose. So if for no other reason, that's surely a motivator. This exercise helps that not-knowing-if-you're-going-to-get-the-key-in-the lock-in-time panic. And when you can even begin to think about it, it helps your sex life, too.

The praying bust lift

What it does: This exercise is fab for toning the boobs as it helps draw in and lift the chest muscles that support your new enlarged breasts, while at the same time working on strengthening your tummy muscles and lower back as you sit on your Swiss ball.

You will need: Your Swiss ball.

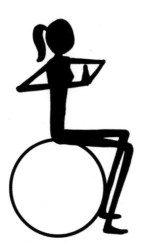

1 Sit on the Swiss ball with your feet flat on the floor. Good posture now, ladies!

2 Keep your belly button pulled in tight to the spine.

3 Extend your arms directly out in front of you and keep them at shoulder height.

4 Bend your arms and press the palms together – as if you were praying (that you don't fall off the Swiss ball!).

5 Hold in those tummy muscles, pressing the palms together. Press for 4 seconds then release. Keep those tummy muscles engaged all the time as this helps to keep your balance.

6 Repeat 12 times. Rest and then get on with another 12.

The tummy toner

What it does: You will be working your deepest abdominal muscles for this simple exercise. This is great to build up strength in your abdominals and your lower back.

You will need: Your Swiss ball.

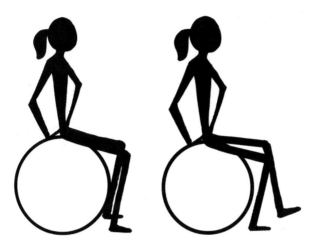

1 Sit on the Swiss ball with your feet flat on the floor and sitting with good posture. Place your hands on your hips.

2 Pull in your navel to your spine and lift one foot just slightly off the floor, only a few centimetres. Hold for a second (at the same time you must engage your abdominals as this is where your balance and strength will come from) then place the foot back down.

3 Repeat with the opposite foot.

4 Aim for 12, rest then repeat another set.

Be nice to yourself

As well as concentrating on your nutrition, make time to think of feeding of a different nature – feeding your soul. You have been through a lot (even though some really capable mothers push through all this with a no-nonsense, bristling efficiency), especially if you are used to feeling in control and suddenly you don't feel in control any more. So be nice to yourself, or you could collapse in a melted pile of exhaustion later down the track – it's a long journey.

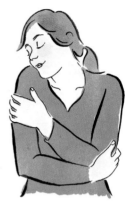

* Take a long bath – grab the moment and don't feel guilty.
* Get someone to come and give you a massage – sometimes student trainees offer discounts. Local training colleges are a good place to go to check out such a thing.
* Take a nap when your baby is resting. You can do the tidying later when you have the energy.
* Read a mag – who cares if it is full of rubbish about celebs? Quite fascinating secretly.
* Go and get your highlights done.
* Do not walk around in your stretchy tracksuit bottoms – even at home.
* Put on your make-up if you are going out.
* Take care of your nutrition – I know I said feed your soul, but you will feel so much better eating great stuff.
* Get some silk pyjamas and a snuggly dressing gown – at least when you are up in the night you'll look beautiful, even if you don't feel it. Nowadays silky fabric washes with the best of them.
* Use my tick lists (see box, opposite).

Your very first tick list

We all want to be perfect and do everything in this book by the book – but don't. The tick lists that run through the book are to reward yourself for things you have focused on – there are points to be won! Doing all of these would, of course, be perfect, but only aim to do four things a day from this tick list – and do them well – and you are a winner.

Exercise

- I did ten 'Squeeze please, Louises' following the sticky note on the mirror in bathroom.
- I held a perfect posture when noticing the sticky note on the kettle when I made a cup of tea.
- I tilted my pelvis ten times when I was in the bathroom.
- I belted up!
- I performed ALL of The Elvis (the King) lives routine.

Nutrition

- I filled a fruit bowl and put it on the table.
- I chucked out all dodgy crisps, ice cream and biscuits.
- I increased the amount of vegetables and fruit that I ate.
- I tried a new fruit or veggie I wouldn't normally have.
- I froze some emergency meals.
- I ate a substantial breakfast.

Be nice to yourself

- I took a nap.
- I had a long bath.
- I read a mag.
- I didn't wear my elephant trousers.
- I put on my make-up.
- I bought a beauty treat.
- I had an early night.

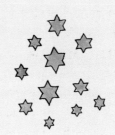

Good news!

* Good news! You may lose 4 to 7kg (9 to 15lb) on the very first day after birth (a mix of baby, placenta and amniotic fluid). The rest is stored fat so that you have enough extra calories for breastfeeding – isn't nature thoughtful?

* Good news! Breastfeeding your baby gobbles up 500–600 extra calories a day.

* Good news! Two hormones called leptin and serotonin work together to put your body in weight-loss mode – no one is quite sure how leptin works exactly but what is certain is that leptin levels stay high throughout pregnancy and that leptin is released by fat tissue and signals the brain to limit fat intake. Leptin levels drop at birth, allowing you to recalibrate your body's 'set point' – your metabolism is working in overdrive to burn more calories than usual to give you extra energy. The serotonin works to control your energy balance and helps keep your appetite in check. So get cracking now with healthy eating – you have the gods on your side.

* Good news! Your tummy may look pretty saggy now, but it will bounce back to where it was.

* Good news! Your uterus contracts during breastfeeding – and helps everything return to shape. These contractions can be quite strong, but keep your chin up, it means your stomach is shrinking.

* Good news! Well not really good news exactly, but if you are feeling really sluggish, treacle tired and really not getting back to where you were – could your thyroid be working below par? Other signs are hair loss and feeling the cold. Worth checking out?

Step away from the scales

Don't always assume that the scales are a true measure of what is going on with the body. If exercise levels are adequate, you may be putting on muscle but losing actual fat, which is what we want, isn't it? Muscle weighs three times more than fat, so concentrate on losing inches even if you are not losing the pounds. I

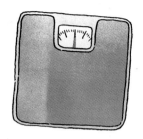

recommend you measure your waist at its narrowest point and your hips at their widest point and do this if you absolutely have to just once a week.

There are lots of ways to determine what you should weigh, but remember that most of these scales are done for average people and can be misleading. For example, body mass index (a scale that looks at mass rather than weight on its own) doesn't take into consideration if you have a lot of muscle. So, obviously don't ignore the indicators of where you should be, but don't feel that you have to live by them either.

Look at the tip on body image on page 188. Loving your body now is the only way you will accept yourself as you are – without all the chat and wishing you were a size 10 – face facts, you aren't. But if you just get on with great nutrition, great exercise and a great attitude, you will be fine. You might want to use the indicator of your clothes to judge whether you have got to your goals, rather than weight alone.

I completely agree with Lucy – give your scales to your worst enemy – they are a curse. Get weighed every so often when you go to the doctors or the gym, but don't live by the scales or you make a pact with the devil!

If you get into the game of weighing yourself every day, then every day becomes a desperate competition with yourself. 'OMYGOD! How could I have put on three pounds in a night?' 'Right,' you declare, 'I am going to take my earrings off, stand on one foot and see if that makes a difference. OK, if I go to the loo, that will knock off a few pounds.' You beat yourself up for the BAD days and stuff your face, because – what does it matter? But when you have actually lost weight, well, you starve yourself all day because you are on the right track – mad logic.

Another game that goes on in your head is to get down to a target weight that, in effect, you have made up. When I played this game, for example, I had to be an 'odd' number on the scales, so I had to be 8 stone 7 and not 8 stone 8 ...

... and, of course, when you get to 8 stone 7, the game is to get to 8 stone 5 ...

... and then that is not really good enough because, in fact, the most ideal weight is 8 stone 3 ...

... Then all your friends start badgering you because you look too thin ... arggh!

So the best thing is, don't even get into those games in the first place. The nutrition programme in this book should liberate you from all that. Please let it. You can allow yourself to be liberated by:

* Blowing up your scales with dynamite – or, better still, giving them to a 'friend'.
* Just cracking on with eating well, doing some exercise and trying to change your attitude.
* If you really can't give up the scales, try putting them on different surfaces.
* Or slightly alter the scale dial to read just a bit lighter, because the scales can't possibly be right. Can they?

A balancing act

Have I got a brilliant no-brainer exercise for you to do or what? All you have to do is be able to stand on one leg. I know that after a long day that can actually prove more difficult than it looks. Why would you want to stand on one leg? Because standing on one leg tones your leg muscles, and gives a little support to your butt muscles – even better, holding the muscles tight increases your metabolism. If you can hold in your tummy at the same time, this helps you to keep your balance, vital to the whole thing. Don't forget to change legs or you will get one toned leg and one flappy one. Oh yes, and keep the knees bent.

Now how easy is that? Feeling better and ready to get down to business? Of course you are!

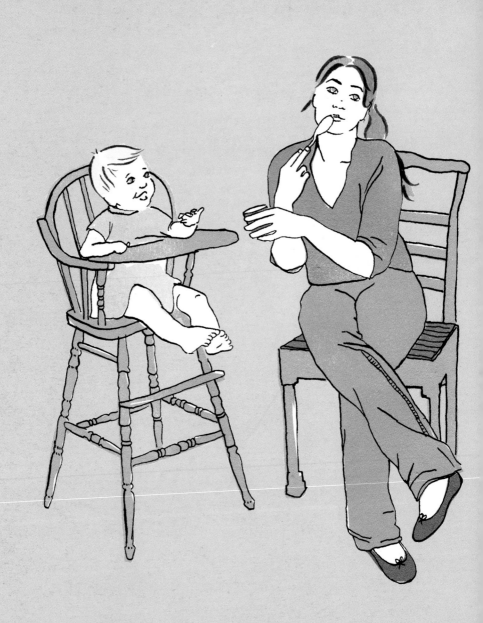

The nutrition bit

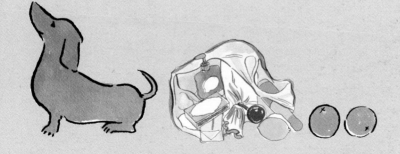

Eat healthily

If I was prescriptive – guess what? I would be giving you a Diet, just like everyone else does. And guess what again? I am sure you have already discovered that you just don't have time to follow diets. They are too much of a schlep – especially with junior in tow. In the old days you could go out shopping for all the 'right' kit and do it all perfectly, but now you have other demands. Without driving yourself crazy, you can no longer be that precise. And calorie counting – we don't do that either – calorie counting long-term doesn't work unless you are very good with maths.

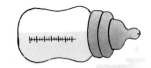

It is important to know that when you start eating right in this way that you are embarking on a journey – you won't be arriving top speed at your destination, but once you're on the road and making a start, step by step, you will get nearer to where you want to be. You will get the results. I have applied the method I am sharing with you with literally thousands of people and so I know it works. Follow this programme and you will be off the slimming diet treadmill and getting on with your life, which is *so* much more important than worrying about your weight all the time.

You don't need to diet to lose weight

Have you noticed how everything these days is over complicated? People want things to be complicated because then it seems as if it is worth it. If the system is too easy, surely it can't be true and can't be working. But remember that people who invent diets are just trying to make money out of you and make it so complicated that you are a prisoner to their system. You have to buy their book – and carry it round with you in your handbag at all times so that every time you feel like eating, you have to check back to see if you are doing the 'right thing' or the 'wrong thing'. The diet only works if you are using their method and if you are unsure how the sacred method works, then you can buy the video, DVD, CD, flashcards, food, calorie counter, exercise pack – and that's a whole lot more money they just made out of you.

The point is that every one of these diet gurus has a part of the truth, but not the whole truth. And following a rigid system disempowers you as a woman. With a twinkle in my eye, I always say that these diets were invented by blokes – blokes who like working on spreadsheets to keep a track of points, calories, goals and other blokey things. We are prisoners to systems to keep us in check. Wouldn't it be powerful if us girls were liberated from the worry of food and that food became something that we really enjoyed without beating ourselves up about it the whole time? How much more time we would have? Tomorrow the world!

Low fat diets

Of course, all diets have an element of truth in them. The no/low fat diets of the Eighties had a point – saturated fat (animal fat) in huge quantities is obviously not a good thing and probably a case of 'a moment on the lips a lifetime on the hips'. The problem is that when you take the fat out of food it tastes really disgusting and so the manufacturers of processed food, in their wisdom, add a whole pile of sugar to products to make them taste even half decent – either real sugar or fake sugars like aspartame. So there might be no fat but there is a load of sugar in it, too.

Low calorie diets

Low calorie diets work too – but boy, do you have to concentrate on the whole thing – either adding up calories or avoiding forbidden foods. And when the day comes that you start eating 'normally' again – like an elastic band that has been stretched and stretched and stretched, when you finally let go and eat a cream bun, you go nuts and can't stop eating 'forbidden' things.

High fibre diets

Then there were the fibre diets, which worked mainly because they were about eating healthier food, but all that fibre without drinking enough water gave people constipation. Also, many of these types of diets relied on wheat as the main source of fibre, and wheat is in a lot of junk food, too. Also eating too much bread can't be good for us either as flour and water, the two major ingredients in bread, make glue. Enough said, I think, don't you?

High protein diets

Then things really swung the other way with Old Dr Atkins and the fear of carbohydrates really took off. Of course, he wasn't the one to actually invent high-protein diets – variations have been around since the ark – but it was Atkins who got rich and famous on it.

Eating loads of protein increases your intake of saturated fats (and all the dangers of that), also all that protein to digest puts your body under a lot of pressure, which the poor old kidneys don't like much.

Atkins thought that the diet worked because the body was producing ketones as a by-product, but in fact all it gave you was bad breath and a bad case of constipation, too. Bliss begins in the bowel and if the bowel is not working properly, you may get all sorts of nasty things down the track. Not worth it.

The glycaemic index

Lately, the glycaemic index (or GI) systems have become all the rage or, even more lately, the GL (glycaemic load). There's nothing new in the GI diets, as Montignac devised his series of books largely based on a GI model in the Eighties. These systems are entirely sensible – lots of fruit and veg, whole foods, some protein, lots of water – real food eaten sensibly. And I love the way that in the front of his book Montignac thanks not one but two cordon bleu chefs. Now that's what I call a diet!

But I come back to the point that these two systems (GI and GL) are still eating plans that trap you in a horrible point-counting black hole. You are not encouraged to think for yourself, but have to buy even more props to keep you on the diet. Before too long you get in a muddle as to which food is high or low GL, or was it GI? Just as you thought you knew how it all worked, you start to have doubts – you'd better check back with the book just in case. 'Blast! The book is in the other handbag. I really don't know what to choose. Yikes!' Then, just when you've got the system down pat, you find out that there are all sorts of exceptions and variations. And for one, such as myself, whose strong point is not maths, calculating all those blessed points is a real pain. I never have enough fingers. Life is really too short. Unless you are absolutely determined and unwavering in your belief in the diet, by day two everything has already gone drastically pear-shaped.

The thing is with dieting and being on a diet, the implication is that one day you won't be on a diet – and then, of course, the pounds slowly but steadily start to pile back on. And so the whole cycle starts again. But read on and you will become a liberated woman, enjoying food for its own sake, safe in the knowledge that by eating healthily, your weight will look after itself.

The easy peasy eating bit and how it works

What we are going to do together is loosely based on the GI system but I have made it really, really easy and in doing this, I'm handing the power back to you, your decisions and you knowing if a food is on the programme or not. There are no lists of good foods and bad foods. There is no point counting, just five really, really simple guidelines that absolutely work – and with only five things to remember, you can keep track of them on the fingers of one hand!

The five rules for healthy eating in a nutshell

1 Keep your energy stable by balancing your blood sugar (sounds complex, but it isn't).
   * Eat food that is thick and fibrous and/or full of protein – this is slow-burn food.
   * Avoid food that is primarily sweet, fluffy and white – this is quick-burn food.

2 Whittle down the wheat. Wheat isn't the only grain in the world, try to replace it with rye, spelt and other grains, such as buckwheat, millet and quinoa. This increases the variation in your diet, so you are not relying on the same old things all the time.

3 Vary your dairy – don't just rely on cow's milk, try other forms of dairy as well, such as goat's and sheep's milk (pasteurised please)

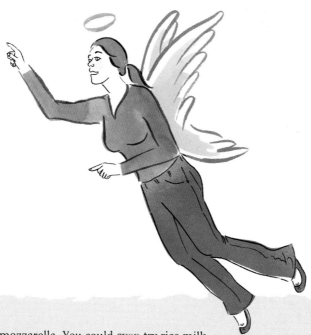

and mozzarella. You could even try rice milk.

Don't over do the dairy – you can get calcium from loads of other sources including green leafy veg.

4 Eat breakfast. You must do this – no arguments – and, if possible, include some protein.

5 Eat like a caveman – this means eating *real* food, organically-produced if possible.

6 Make up your own rule. I know I said there were five rules, but this is one for you to make up for yourself if you want to. It is a wild-card rule. You might, for example, decide to eat only a handful portion of low-burn carbohydrates at your evening meal as opposed to a great big plateful. Or you might want it as an exercise rule or to build it around portion size or drinking.

Rule 1: Keep your energy stable by balancing your blood sugar

You must keep your blood sugar balanced to avoid crashes of energy. This sounds more complicated than it is.

We have about a teaspoon of sugar (glucose) in the blood at any one time. Sugar is our fuel and powers our system, but too much of a good thing is not necessarily wonderful. In fact, too much sugar is positively not a good thing at all. The body is always trying to maintain a state of balance and has complicated feedback systems to keep everything in check. The blood sugar is lowered by a hormone called insulin, which allows the cells of your body to open up and 'put away' the sugar. Therefore, if we eat foods that produce too much sugar and raise the blood sugar too high, our bodies panic, pump in a lot of insulin and the blood sugar is rapidly lowered. *Slump!*

At this point you say to yourself, 'Hmm, I feel a nice chocolate biscuit calling.'

Because that chocolate biscuit is quite sweet, up shoots the blood sugar and in comes that hormone insulin to lower the sugar in the blood. You have a rollercoaster of blood sugar, instead of a nice even, consistent energy supply.

Stimulants will also raise and crash blood sugar (think caffeine or nicotine – surely not still smoking?). What I should just mention is that insulin's other job is to store fat – so if you have too many of these big rushes of insulin, caused by a rush of sugar, your body is going to decide to store some fat and this fat loves to deposit itself around your tummy and hips.

Avoid sweet foods

Some food burns quickly and some burns slowly in the system. Foods that are sweet are going to put more sugar in your system than foods that burn slowly. Any food (pretty much) that you put in your mouth that is sweet is going to affect your blood sugar. So although some sweet foods have other benefits (like they contain vitamins and minerals), from a blood sugar point of 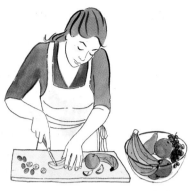 view, they are not such a good idea. A good example could be tropical fruit – great for all sorts of other reasons – but quite sweet. Therefore choose the British fruits like, apples, pears, damsons, cherries, and berries rather than mangoes, pineapples and bananas.

Avoid fluffy and white foods

Food that is fluffy and/or white tends to be food that has been processed. The more processed a food, the higher the burn. Food that is white is quite often starchy food and – guess what, folks? – starch is sugar.

Fluffy means light food, which includes:

* White rice
* Puffed rice cereals
* Candy floss
* Bread (which seems to have a lot of air in it these days).

And white food that has been processed includes:

* Pasta: go for the wholegrain version
* Rice: go for the brown version
* Bread: go for a wheat-free version, such as rye breads, as these breads tend to be made in an artisan way, are heavier and less full of rubbish. These days there are some excellent rye breads that are not the worthy pumpernickel types of yore. Try Village Bakery (www.village-bakery.com) Borodinsky bread, which is fabulous, or www.stamp-collection.co.uk for wheat-free breads generally.

Go for thick and fibrous and/or protein

If you want your blood sugar to remain stable, you have to eat foods that are heavy and dense and thick – these foods take longer to digest and therefore the sugar goes into the blood stream in a more sustained way. A good example of a thick, fibrous food would be the humble lentil. If you took a single lentil and put it under a microscope you would see that it is very dense and fibrous with no air holes. If you had a machine that could enlarge the lentil into a giant lentil the size of a rock, you would notice that it would be very heavy too. A lentil also happens to be full of protein. So, a lentil would be an ideal slow-burn food.

Natural muesli is a heavy food as compared to Rice Crispies. Anything brown or with a skin on it is going to be heavier than the white version of it (brown rice, brown pasta, whole, unprocessed foods.) Most green vegetables are going to be fibrous and fruit with skin on it is going to be higher in fibre than the peeled version. So far so good?

Lower the blood sugar

If you want to lower the effect a food is going to have on the blood sugar, then add either protein or fibre.

* If you had an apple (which is a bit sweet, *but* it has skin so is fibrous) and ate it with a small handful of nuts, which are protein (any natural nuts such as cashews, Brazils, almonds, hazelnuts, or walnuts), your blood sugar would not rise so fast.
* If you had a baked potato and hollowed out some of the middle (white and fluffy) and added in some protein – organic, no sugar baked beans or some cottage cheese, for example – you would lower the burn.

Things like carrots get a bad press for being sweet once cooked but when was the last time you had an entire plate of cooked carrots? Once you add fibre and a bit of protein the burn will be sufficiently lowered – so just don't worry about it.

The slow and fast burn game

Here are the rules: take a look at each of the foods and say whether you think they are either fast burners (i.e. white, sweet or fluffy) or slow burners (i.e. thick, fibrous or protein). There are 500 points available (non-redeemable) if you guess correctly. The answers are given at the end of the list.

1   Fruit juice
2   All whole grains – stuff like brown rice, real, thick porridge (but they musn't be processed)
3   Quinoa (whacky South American grains)
4   Tropical fruit
5   Inside of a baked potato
6   Meat, fish, chicken, nuts and tofu
7   Candy
8   Biscuits
9   Chocolate
10 Potatoes
11 All green veg
12 Other brightly-coloured stuff, such as peppers
13 Cauliflower
14 Chickpeas, lentils, pulses and beans
15 Rye breads or real artisan heavy wholewheat bread
16 Mueslis made with whole grains
17 Honey
18 Real, natural yoghurt with added English, sourer-type fruit

1   Fast (sweet)
2   Slow (fibrous)
3   Slow (protein)
4   Fast (sweet)
5   Fast (fluffy)
6   Slow (protein)
7   Fast (sweet, fluffy and white)
8   Fast (sweet and white)
9   Fast (sweet)
10 Slow (white and sometimes fluffy – go for sweet potatoes, which although have sweet in the title are actually very fibrous)
11 Slow (fibrous)
12 Slow (fibrous)
13 Slow (fibrous, even though it's white – it's dense and not processed)
14 Slow (protein and fibrous)
15 Slow (fibrous)
16 Slow (fibrous)
17 Fast (sweet)
18 Slow (protein and fruit is fibrous)

Don't be afraid of carbs

Somewhere out there in the darkness of the deepest darkest forest is the spooky carbohydrate monster – this monster makes you put on weight by just looking you right between the eyes. Thwack! A love handle is formed and only the protein angel can save you from this wickedness – hmmm, I don't think so.

The thing is, we have apparently developed a fear of all known carbohydrates and people don't really seem to know the difference between the crappy old carbohydrates – the refined type with no vitamins, minerals and no fibre – and the great carbohydrates that give you energy and goodness. They are all tarred with the same brutally wicked brush. Everything, sometimes including fruit and veg, is all lumped together in one manifestation of evilness. This is plainly quite bonkers as fruit and veg and whole grains give you a helpful dollop of nutrients.

Don't get to the desperation stage where you will try anything to shift poundage – fatty meats and cheeses are not the way forward, whatever they tell you in the best-selling books – the only thing you will be successful at is having a constipated bottom, smelly breath and no friends. Carbs give you energy and boy do you need energy when you are the mother of a newborn – starches and sugars are your body's primary source of glucose, providing fuel for your brain, your blood and your nervous system.

Primarily, good carbs are things that are covered in skin, like brown rice, other whole grains such as rye, barley and oats, sweet potatoes and leafy green vegetables. In just a few days that constipation will have disappeared on a diet full of fruit and veg and whole grains, and you will be back on the invite list for the party set, now that your breath is sweet again.

Rules 2: Whittle down the wheat

Everything in moderation, including moderation itself, but it is absolutely amazing how much wheat we can potentially shove in to our mouths in one day. The following menu is a real diet that I took from a real patient I saw yesterday. By anyone's standards this is not varied enough.

Breakfast
Weetabix with milk (clue in the title)
Latte coffee (dairy)
Apple juice (sweet, while we are at it)

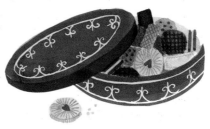

Snack
4 rich tea biscuits (wheat)
Latte and biscuit (dairy and wheat)
Strawberry yoghurt (dairy)

Lunch
Cheddar cheese sandwich with tomatoes (wheat and dairy)

Snack
Lots of mini-chocolate rolls and polished off kid's dinner of pasta shapes (wheat)

Dinner
Pasta with pesto and green salad (wheat, dairy - Parmesan cheese - well done for including a salad!)

Once you learn to look around for other alternatives to wheat:

✳ You first realise that there is a *massive* choice available to you.
✳ Second, you realise how much rubbish food contains wheat.

It doesn't take much to vary the diet until it becomes second nature.

Wheat is present in a wide variety of foods, from the obvious sources such as bread, cakes and biscuits to sauces, seasonings and many processed foods, and it is one of the most commonly eaten allergens in the UK.

An intolerance or sensitivity to wheat is a common cause of tiredness, loss of concentration and digestive problems. Stop to consider how often it is eaten, possibly at every meal; wheat-based cereal or toast, sandwich for lunch and pasta in the evening, and that's not including any biscuits, cakes or snacks during the day.

Gluten contained in wheat is a sticky substance that is capable of reducing the absorption of nutrients in susceptible people. In fact, the mixture of processed white wheat flour and water is sticky enough to be used as wallpaper paste – this is certainly not the effect that we want to be happening in our stomachs. In some individuals, wheat gluten can act as a brain irritant.

It is this glue-like property that makes wheat so difficult to digest, requiring a great deal of energy to do so. For this reason, it is often found that by eliminating wheat, energy levels increase dramatically, thus leaving more energy for the body to repair and heal itself. Remember that wheat-free does not always mean gluten-free.

Alternative grains

Flours: Barley, buckwheat, chickpea, maize, potato, rice, quinoa, rye, tapioca, millet and chestnut flour and soya

Crackers: Corn cakes, oatcakes, rice cakes, rye crackers or crispbreads, savoury biscuits (Village Bakery make gluten-free ones)

Pasta: Corn, millet, spelt, buckwheat, kamut or vegetable varieties. Try Mother Hemp Spelt and Hemp pasta, it tastes like regular pasta (go to www.motherhemp.com)

Whole grains: Barley, buckwheat, kamut, millet, rye, quinoa, brown rice, oats and corn

Lunch alternatives

- Jacket potato with a protein filling (cottage cheese, tuna, egg) and some salad
- Soup (check the ingredients if not home-made) with crackers or wheat-free bread and tuna or beans for some protein and more substance
- Mixed salad with nuts, seeds, apple and avocado
- Bean salads with olive oil, lemon and herbs – try parsley, coriander or chives
- Corn, oat or rice cakes with hummus, nut butter, vegetables, fish pâté (check for wheat content), avocado, cottage cheese
- Bean burgers, tofu sausages (check the ingredients), grilled or poached fish with salad

Rule 3: Vary your dairy

This is the same story really – we can tot up a huge amount of dairy points in a day if we are not careful; just remember to vary the type of dairy you have so that you get a broad spectrum of nutrients. Think how many cappuccinos some people main-line. Relying on one or two types of food is not a good definition of a varied diet.

There is also a lot of chat and beating of the nutritional bongo drums about dairy generally. Is dairy food the super duper wonder food that we were led to believe, even if we were all brought up on it? The comfort of the milk moustache with the large glass of milk before bedtime? We are the only mammals, as far as I am aware, to suckle another big mammal's milk into adulthood and the more milk you drink, 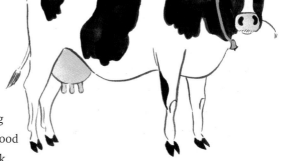 the higher the level of a hormone called IGF-1 (insulin-like growth factor) there is in your blood. The higher the IGF-1, the higher the risk for breast cancer. In rural China, breast cancer is a relatively unknown, while in the UK, the rates are one person in eight. Makes you think? And before you say it, there are plenty of other good sources of calcium – leafy green veg for one (see the box, right).

Alternative sources of calcium

* Dark green leafy vegetables – spinach, kale, cabbage, watercress
* Nuts and seeds (especially sesame)
* Soya
* Sardines
* Parsley
* Pulses
* Prunes

Rule 4: Eat breakfast

Breakfast means breaking the fast. Over night the levels of sugar in the blood drop – so if you have a sugary, sweet, light or fluffy breakfast, the blood sugar rises steeply for that inevitable crash. Normally at around 11am. Masses of people say to me that when they eat breakfast they actually feel more hungry and not less – so they are often tempted to skip breakfast altogether. The reason that you feel hungrier is because you are eating all the wrong foods! The sweet, fluffy and white types of food will make you feel starving. The fluffy foods are white toast with jam and orange juice, Rice Crispies, cereal with loads of sugar, etc.

Instead, you need a dense, thick fibrous breakfast and the best choice would be:

* Porridge (proper jumbo oats) with rice milk and berries, but be careful that you don't compensate by scattering on a mound of sugar to make it taste better.
* Wheat-free muesli (only wheat free because they tend to be made without sugar and also have a variation of grains).
* Eggs: boiled, scrambled (you don't need butter or milk, just scramble the eggs in a non-stick pan), poached, omelette – with spinach, tomatoes, asparagus or sugar snap peas.

- Kippers.
- Kedgeree made with brown rice.
- Sardines on toast with tomatoes (even from a tin)
  – I know this one is a big ask!
- Pasteurised goat's cheese/mozzarella and
  tomatoes on toast with watercress.
- Cashew nut butters with rye toast.

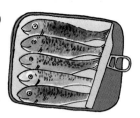

Rule 5: Eat like a caveman

I don't really mean eat like an actual caveman – all those hairy
mammoths and scurrying around looking under rocks for worms.
Think of your nails, for a start. I do, however, mean the idea of
eating real food that hasn't been processed. Cavemen had to hunt
for their food, fish for it, kill it, skin it, build
a fire, cook on it. Or they had to grow
it, wait a really long time and then
harvest it, grind it up, cook it,
mash it. What an adventure
food must have been way
back then.

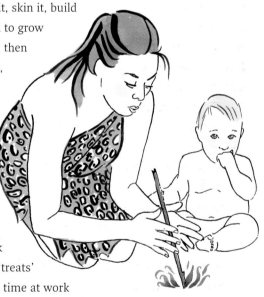

Think how easy it is
to get our hands on food
now. We just have to head
up the road to the local
supermarket and fill the
trolley. It is tempting to stack
the trolley full of all sorts of 'treats'
(after all, we have had a hard time at work
and surely must deserve one of Mr Kipling's 'delicious'
cakes?). We may think that a Kipling's cake will hit the spot, but
our bodies disagree – they haven't evolved much. In fact, our
bodies' reaction and requirement of food hasn't changed since
we were swinging through the trees, but our modern food has
dramatically changed – and to think this has more or less happened

in the last 40 years or so. Even when I was a kid in the Seventies there really wasn't that much junk food – Fray Bentos Pies (delicious by the way, but I can't think what can be in them), and peas and fish fingers. Oh, and Angel Delight. Sheer poison.

I am sure after the depravation of the war years, all this instant, cheap food must have seemed too good to be true. The truth is, it is too good to be true. Our bodies, although jolly clever, haven't adapted to eating all the rubbish we throw at them. They are not used to eating the sweet, white and fluffy foods that most junk foods consist of – and everyone is scratching their heads trying to work out why the Western nations are turning into huge, lardy fatty-puffs – eating food that is not real food, that is how it's happened. We have turned our bodies over to food scientists who want to prolong shelf life, or the advertisers who want to make money out of us. We are no longer making our own decisions. When you eat real food, it is really difficult to eat a highly calorific diet – vegetables, fruit, whole grains, fish and chicken and pulses are not naturally highly calorific and they are very filling. If you eat junk food, of course you have to count calories or pretty quickly you will massively exceed what you need to eat in a day.

In the West we may have all the calories we require, but do we have all the nutrients we need? We might even be malnourished (not enough vitamins and minerals). This rule is therefore about eating real food, food that you can recognise as food. Food that doesn't have all sorts of words on the label beginning with 'x' and are more than three syllables. Food that smells like food. Generally also food that can be cooked and made into something – rather than food that is already something as soon as you get it home from the shops. A drag it may be, but otherwise you will pay for it.

Rule 6: Make up your own rule

This rule is not a real rule at all because it is your choice as to what you do with it. You don't even have to make a rule if you don't want. You can make this one fit in with where you are at the moment. My rule six, for example, is: 'I only drink champagne', which is great because it stops me drinking lukewarm wine at a party but if there is a special occasion, I am really up for celebrating.

I am hi-jacking this rule also as the 'blindingly obvious rule'. You are too intelligent to really think that foods lathered in sugar, ice cream, fat, treacle, loads of high-fat dressings or marshmallows are healthy foods or magic foods that don't count. Also, while a little of what you fancy does you good – seconds and thirds of chocolate or loads of red wine (whatever the French Red Wine Marketing Bureau has told you about the benefits of antioxidants), vats of butter and huge helpings generally will make you fat.

If you are casting around for a rule number six, one of the best things you can do is to do the following: 'include a handful of low-burn carbohydrates with my evening meal'. Instead of having a huge great big plateful of the supporting carb with the evening meal, have a smaller handful of low-burn carbs. Slow burning carbs are things with skin on them, which are fibrous. Not white and fluffy foods like mashed potatoes.

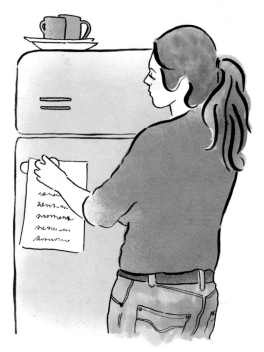

Examples of slower burning carbohydrates are:

✳ Sweet potatoes	✳ Bulgar
✳ Brown basmati rice	✳ Chickpeas
✳ Buckwheat	✳ Lentils
✳ Whole grain pasta	✳ Beans
✳ Barley	✳ Sprouted seeds

Other whole grains would be fabulous, too, including the high protein seed quinoa.

If you are breastfeeding, you must have a goodly amount of slow burning carbs – you are burning 500 extra calories a day and need the energy. The rest of you can choose either to have a handful of slow burn carbs or not to have the *big* carbs, which is my terminology for:

✳ Pizza
✳ Pasta
✳ Potatoes and other starchy veg, such as parsnips
✳ Bread
✳ White rice

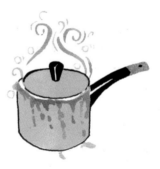

Clue to you breastfeeding ladies

If you are breastfeeding and not eating enough, you will be losing weight too quickly – eat more. If you are starving most of the time – and eating the 'right' kind of kit – you are not eating enough either.

Last word

Don't drive yourself nuts. This is not a diet – so it means that 80 per cent of the time follow the rules and 20 per cent of the time blow a big raspberry at the rules and do what you like! Remember that although it may look like I am saying 'no' in some of the rules, actually all I am asking you to do is to say 'no' to 80 per cent of them. For the remaining 20 per cent have yourself some fun. Of course, the more you do, the better the result, but don't pull yourself too tight or one day, you will want to break out, diet style. A blip is just a blip. Don't beat yourself up and don't worry if you go veering off-piste – it happens. Even to nutritionists.

In this system, I deliberately want you to get the spirit of the law and not the letter of the law. In this way you learn to relax about food and let all your choices 'be OK', as our American cousins might say. If you go by the letter of the law and are worrying too much about the details, you are probably getting obsessed. There are plenty of diets out there that will help you get obsessed but I don't plan to add to them. Once you get the hang of the above you can do this for the rest of your life. How liberating is that?

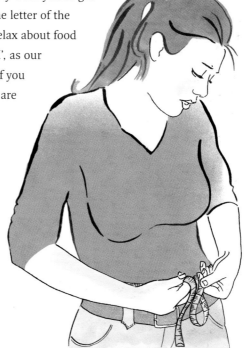

Other stuff

Alcohol

I am not your mother and therefore I am not going to give you a
huge lecture, letting you make up your own mind on this one. Let it
be said, however, that you are a braver woman than me if you can
handle drinking and a young baby. Of course you know if you are
breastfeeding loads of alcohol is not a great idea
anyway – two to three glasses a week max. It
doesn't take a size nine hat to realise that if you
drink, it is better done after the baby's last feed –
so the alcohol has dissipated before feeding in the
night. Alcohol weakens any promises you make to
yourself about being on any kind of health kick.
That's all I am going to say.

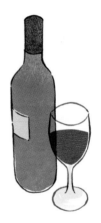

Oh, and you think that the alcohol will make
you feel better but, in fact, it just makes you feel
crap and it depletes your B vits and so you will
actually feel more stressed than ever, because B
vits give you a healthy nervous system.

Vitamins and minerals

Vibrant vitamin A

There are lots of vital vitamins that you need – especially if you are
breastfeeding. Vitamin A is really important for proper growth of
your baby and it is also good for healthy skin and a strong immune
system – and why wouldn't you want that?

Vitamin A is a fat-soluble vitamin found in animal foods (retinol)
and in some vegetables (betacarotene, which is especially rich in
orange vegetables like sweet potatoes). Foods that contains good
quantities of vitamin A are:

* Apricots
* Asparagus
* Cabbage
* Carrots
* Liver, although best not eaten if you are actually pregnant
* Papayas
* Squash
* Sweet potatoes
* Tangerines
* Tomatoes
* Watercress

Warning!
If you decide to take vitamin supplements, then don't take more than 3,000mcg or 10,000iu of retinal. If you are of childbearing age, too much retinal can lead to abnormalities in pregnancy for the baby. In addition, too much vitamin A can be stored in the liver and mega amounts can even be toxic.

Vital vitamin B

B vitamins are great for energy and stress. And, wow, do you need that with a wee baby in tow. B vits (B1–B6, B12, biotin and, of course, the famous folic acid – remember that from your pregnancy days?) help our nervous system, the brain development in a growing child and skin and hair, too. They are found in the following foods:

* Bananas (B6)
* Broccoli
* Cabbage
* Chicken
* Cottage cheese (B12)
* Eggs
* Lamb
* Nuts and seeds (folic acid)
* Salmon (B3)
* Sardines
* Squash
* Tomatoes
* Watercress

If you go down the supplement route (see page 69), always take B vits within a multi-vitamin or within a B-complex because the B group of vitamins work together.

Vibrant vitamin C

When we were gibbons swinging through the trees, scoffing fruit on the way, we probably had so much vitamin C that we didn't know what to do with it. In fact, we are one of the few mammals that don't manufacture vitamin C ourselves, in our bodies.

Now listen up – I hope you ate enough in pregnancy because vitamin C goes towards collagen, which is important for nice elasticated skin. Vit C is also a good anti-ageing vit and if you don't want to be prey to masses of colds and infections this winter, make sure you are getting enough.

Vibrant vitamin D

There is exciting chat on the nutritional bongo drums about vitamin D – could it be an important vitamin in cancer prevention and are we getting enough?

Eat loads of eggs, herring, mackerel, oysters and salmon, which are good sources.

Vibrant vitamin E

This is a vitamin that helps protect you from ageing, keeping your cells supple – worth getting enough of?

To ensure you do, eat loads of beans, peas, salmon, sardines, sesame seeds, sunflower seeds and sweet potatoes.

The mighty minerals

Zinc

Zinc is the truly mighty mineral and your wee babe is 'stealing' a lot of your supplies through your breast milk. Making sure you have enough could be the difference between cheerfulness and being down in the dumps. Getting plentiful supplies has a huge effect on mental wellbeing and energy levels – and it's good for your hair, too.

You might want to take a multi-vitamin as well (see page 69) – usually a good one will have about 15mg of zinc but you could take up to 25mg. Zinc helps the immune system to function at the top of its game as well ... all in all, making sure you have enough of it is a jolly good idea to stop you getting run down. The following foods contain it:

* Almonds
* Green peas
* Haddock
* Lamb chops
* Oats
* Pecans

* Rye
* Shrimps
* Turnips (now you know)
* Whole wheatgrain

Calcium

We all know that calcium is good for bones and teeth, but it's also good for a healthy heart and nervous system. You might worry that you aren't getting enough if you aren't chuggerlugging the dairy, but rest assured that as long as you are eating loads of other sources of calcium and perhaps are taking a multi-vitamin too, you will be well stocked with calcium – especially if you are eating your greens. In addition to dairy, other sources of calcium are:

* Almonds
* Cabbage
* Cooked dried beans
* Globe articokes
* Leafy green veg
  (which also contains
  magnesium to help
  absorb the calcium)
* Meat
* Parsley
* Poultry

Getting the most from your food
* Don't overcook food as it spoils the vitamins and minerals.
* Eat wholefoods – those that haven't been mucked about with.
* If possible, eat local, fresh and organic.
* Eat the whole fruit rather than pre-prepared fruit you can buy in supermarkets.

Magnesium

Magnesium helps muscles relax and is good for your energy production, too. Eat loads of:

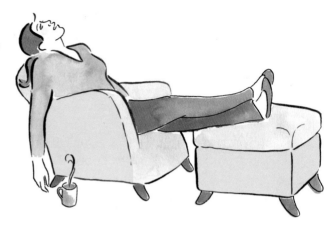

* Brazil nuts
* Buckwheat flour
* Cashews
* Cooked beans
* Garlic
* Peas
* Pecans
* Potato skins
* Raisins
* Wheat germ

Iron

If you are feeling really knackered, ask the doctor to give you a test for low iron – the symptoms are lethargy, pale skin and a sore tongue. You can also eat:

* Almonds
* Cashews
* Cooked dried beans
* Dried prunes
* Parsley
* Pecans
* Pumpkin
* Raisins
* Red meat
* Sesame seeds

Selenium

This is one of the great minerals that helps us have a healthy immune system – it helps protect us against damage from pollution and is found in:

* Cabbage
* Chicken
* Cod
* Courgettes
* Herring
* Molasses
* Mushrooms

Chromium

Chromium is one of the minerals that helps balance your blood sugar and reduce cravings. It is found in:

* Apples
* Brewer's yeast
* Butter
* Chicken
* Cornmeal
* Eggs
* Green peppers
* Lamb chops
* Rye bread

Manganese

Us nutritional types say, 'manganese sore knees' partly because it rhymes but mostly because you need manganese for healthy bones, cartilage, tissues and nerves. It is found in:

* Brown rice
* Cereals
* Nuts
* Pulses
* Watercress

Iodine

Iodine helps to maintain thyroid function, which is really important as the thryoid is your body's thermostat and it is better for weight loss and energy if it is working properly. Find it in:

* Chicken
* Cod
* Haddock
* Mackerel
* Pilchards
* Plaice
* Yoghurt

Supplementing your diet

While we are on the subject of vitamins and minerals – make sure that you supplement your diet with a really good multi-vitamin, especially if you are breastfeeding, because your baby is gobbling up a lot of resources. Good ones are the Pre-natal Pack (Biotics) – yes, I know it says 'Pre' but it is great for post natal, too. Available through your friendly nutritional therapist.

Foods to increase

Bio yoghurt

Or live yoghurt. Naturally occurring cultures can enhance digestion and maintain a healthy gut flora and bowel function. Live sheep's and goat's milk yoghurt are available for those who cannot tolerate cow's milk products.

Fresh fruits and vegetables

Choose a range of varieties and colours for a range of nutrients. These foods naturally contain carotenoids, which are powerful blood and liver cleansers, beneficial for the skin and respiratory tract. Fruits and vegetables are a great source of antioxidants that help protect the cells from environmental and internal damage.

Eat: Apricots, broccoli, carrots, cauliflower, mangetout, peas, peppers, squash, swedes and tomatoes.

Apples

A good source of vitamin C, magnesium and pectin. Pectin binds to toxins and heavy metals, such as lead (pollution) and cadmium (cigarettes), and it can also help to reduce high 'bad' cholesterol.

Berries

These generally have a lower sugar content than tropical fruits and are especially high in antioxidants.

Eat: Blackberries, black and redcurrants, blueberries, cherries, cranberries, raspberries and strawberries.

Citrus fruits

These are also good sources of vitamin C as well as bioflavonoids (which enhance the action of vitamin C) and betacarotene.

Eat: Lemons, limes, oranges and grapefruit.
But avoid if you suffer from irritable bowel syndrome, endometriosis, dermatitis, arthritis or psoriasis.

Tropical fruits

These are often grown in mineral-rich soils so contain good levels of minerals. Pineapple and papaya contain enzymes that can help with protein digestion. Remember to eat them with a little protein, such as nuts, seeds or yoghurt, in order to keep blood sugar levels stable.

Eat: Guava, kiwis, lychees, mangoes, melon, papaya and pineapple.

Green leafy vegetables

These foods are good replacements for carbohydrates as they are fibrous, filling, full of nutrients and easy to digest. Cruciferous vegetables (those that grow in a 'crossover' pattern) are thought to be anti-carcinogenic.

Eat: Broccoli, Brussels sprouts, cabbage, endive, kale, spinach and watercress.

Onions, garlic and leeks

These act as natural antibiotics, help to reduce excessive blood clotting and lower the total cholesterol count while increasing the HDL cholesterol ('good' cholesterol). Their action as pre-biotics (feeding the 'friendly' bacteria) can have a beneficial effect on the digestive system.

Legumes and pulses

These are an excellent source of fibre, B vitamins and protein. Lentils provide iron and all types of beans can help to reduce cholesterol, regulate colon function and help to control blood sugar levels. Soya beans and soya products contain isoflavones that can help to balance hormones.

Eat: Borlotti beans, butter beans, cannellini beans, chickpeas, haricot beans and lentils.
Avoid lentils and pulses if you suffer from gout as they may aggravate the condition.

Nori and wakame seaweeds

Eat these for their selenium and iodine content. They also contain alginates, which help detoxify the body. They can be added to stews and soups or to beans and pulses during cooking.

Nuts and seeds

Raw, unroasted and unsalted only. Try not to exceed more than a small handful per day as they do have a high fat content, but they contain large amounts of essential fatty acids. Add them to cereals, salads, rice and grain dishes, or anywhere you fancy an extra crunch. Nuts and seeds also contain calcium, magnesium, zinc and fibre.

Eat: Almonds, Brazils, cashews, hazelnuts, pecans, walnuts and flax, pumpkin, sesame and sunflower seeds.

Oily fish

Essential omega-3 fatty acids contained in oily fish can help protect the cardiovascular system and they have strong anti-inflammatory properties, which may improve a number of skin and joint disorders. Where possible, choose wild fish if not organic farmed varieties, as these may be lower in antibiotics and other additives.

Eat: Anchovies, herrings, kippers, mackerel, salmon, sardines, pilchards, trout and fresh tuna.

Organic chicken, lamb, pheasant and venison

Good sources of protein that are free from antibiotics and hormones.

Organic free-range eggs

A good source of protein, B vitamins, zinc and iron and essential fats. The saturated fat content of eggs depends on what the chickens were fed, hence eggs from organic free-range chickens have a lower saturated fat content.

Whole grains

These are good sources of fibre, B vitamins, chromium and trace elements; they provide a slow, sustained release of energy that helps to keep blood sugar level stable.

Eat: Amaranth, barley, brown basmati rice, buckwheat, kamut, millet, oats, quinoa, rye and spelt.

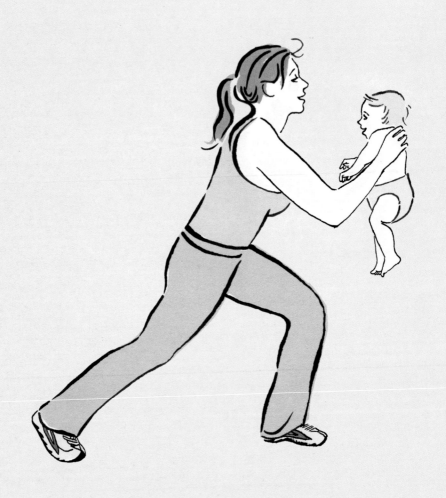

The exercise
and putting it
all together bit

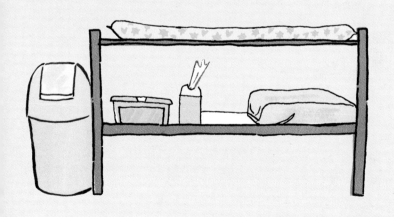

The Day of Reckoning beckons . . .

Right! This is the morning you go and give your old jeans a strict talking to. They still look like they shrunk in the wash (at least nine months ago), but either they'll have to change or you will and maybe it had better be you; they appear awfully stubborn just at the moment. So, you give in – tomorrow is the day to start to get a grip and follow some of this nutrition and exercise stuff. Nothing too strenuous mind, just enough to show those jeans who's boss around here.

Some mental preparation seems to be required before diving into this. Getting into shape is something you've talked enough about, for goodness sake – even in the hospital between the gas and air. And giving yourself a mental bashing for not getting started has become an Olympic sport – in fact, you have been going for gold.

But hang on just a minute. Hasn't your entire lifestyle changed? Until that stork paid a little visit, weren't you in charge of both your life and your body? He just flapped off leaving you to it and didn't even leave the instruction manual. It's been a *huge* adjustment. So, first give yourself a medal – after all, you've got the chest to pin it on. You survived. Well done. Now get a piece of paper and start writing a list of what you will need to do in preparation for tomorrow.

Check out who's on side

You are the managing director of this family – but have you got your lovely, supportive partner on side for your fitness mission? This is going to be key when the going gets tough. It is really easy for you to put everyone else's needs above yours and suddenly you find that the exercise you were going to make time for has gone out of the window. So talk to him and tell him you are serious. You could point out (sweetly) that maybe Wednesdays and Fridays are your 'health nights' and would he be in charge of the baby monitor for a few hours.

Look around and see who else you could recruit. Your mum? Neighbours? Friends? Could you stretch to paying for a couple of hours help? Give yourself a really good chance of making this more than a feeble attempt by allowing yourself some time.

Pair up

Subtly find out if any other mother wants to team up with you and be your buddy in your mission to reclaim your trousers. Tread carefully, though, as, 'You need to do something urgently about the size of your tummy' won't win you the friends or support you are looking for. Instead, she might just go for, 'I am doing this ridiculous health kick thingy, and I know you don't need to, but I was just wondering ... will you please do it with me for a bit of moral support?'

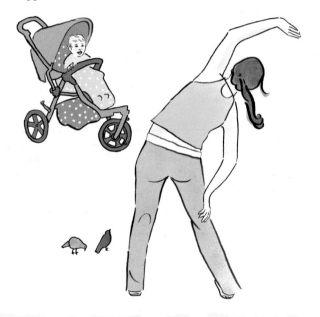

Never start a new resolution on a Monday!
It is far too depressing and you will have given up by midweek. Start on a Wednesday with less pressure. At the weekend you will hopefully have some help with the baby, enabling you to have time to run around the entire park five times. Actually, make that walk – once. But anyway, you will get some you-time.

Kit up

Have you got the right kit? The last exercise clothes you had were designed for a stick. If you can run to it money-wise, go and get something really nice and inspiring – not the great big old grey elephant-like pants and baggy 'am I in here?' T-shirt you were planning on wearing. Act sexy, alluring and wonderful now – don't wait. Don't forget good shoes, and above all a decent sports bra – otherwise all that bouncing up and down will put you off.

And while you are at, treat yourself to a new bag of make-up. If you see that snooty glamorous blonde at mother and play group one more time in her flawless foundation, you will no doubt kill her with your bare hands. How does someone get to be that perfect? Not the slightest signs of re-growth at the roots. Maybe it is genetic.

Get out the dosh – buy the stuff in – even if it does cost a few pence to get all of it. Chuck out all the crappy stuff. Look, you can't expect to be perfectly organised all the time, but having the stuff to hand is going to help a whole lot, believe me.

Pat yourself on the back

Write all the things you are good at on another piece of paper. Do it now! Even the small things count. For example, you have been up all night, but still managed not to be crabby this morning, is a good start.

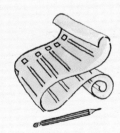

Are you ready? A tick list

☐ The night before, lay out all your baby's clothes. If you have weaned your baby, work out what you are going to give him to eat – can it be something you are eating?

☐ If you are making bottles as opposed to breastfeeding, make up the bottles for the day in advance and put them in the fridge.

☐ Have you got the right exercise gear?

☐ Do you know what you are going to wear?

☐ For your food, make sure you have the basics and if you have decided to follow the sample menus on pages 93–7, then make sure that you have got all the necessary food for those, too.

☐ Revise the six nutrition principles (see page 48) – better still, tattoo them on your arm. Only kidding. Write them down on an index card and keep them in your pocket.

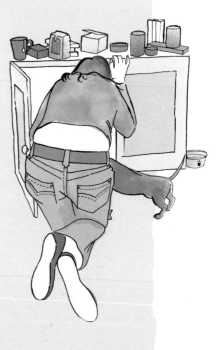

And finally . . .

Just to let you know, I have laid out the exercises only in a *suggested* way, this is definitely not a prescription – you need to be highly flexible so that you can make it work around your baby. Do not attempt to do the routines to the letter because your baby will sleep at different times and feed at different times. Some babies are just really 'good' and some are just really not. A mother I met the other day coming back from playgroup had had her toddler in a flaming tantrum for two-and-a-half hours until she ran his head under a cold tap. Look – she was desperate. She was in tears.

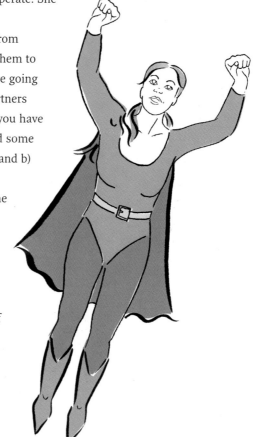

So, just get some ideas from these pages and then adapt them to suit your life. Some of you are going to get great support from partners and some are not – some of you have mums who can take over and some mums (mine), a) live in Italy and b) do not like small children.

Don't stand there with the book in your hand at all times, wondering what to do next. Adapt, adapt, adapt this to *your* unique, wonderful life!

Today is the beginning of the rest of your life.

So let's get cracking.

How the exercise programme works

In this part of the book I have designed an effective fitness plan for you to be a deliciously yummy mummy in no time.

Are you sure this is fun, Lucy?

Fun is our middle name in this – you'll see.

Each week is different, so you will never get bored and at the end of the programme you can then pick and create your own variations from the exercises you have learnt, to maintain your new healthy physique.

I have created the exercises especially as you need to avoid certain moves that cause over stretching because you will still have the hormone relaxin floating around your system for potentially six months after giving birth (for more on relaxin, see page 106).

I have also designed the exercises to focus on toning, lifting up and pulling in all the areas to give you a fabulous hourglass shape. They will tone your arms, nip in the waist and lift your butt.

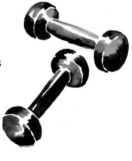

Interesting ... now how does it work?

Well, we are going to be focusing on two forms of exercise. The first being the aerobic type in the form of power pram walking, which will dramatically increase your energy, improve your cardiovascular health and burn off any extra baby weight.

The other is essential toning. It's time to recondition those muscles that have been mega stretched over the past nine months. Toning gets everything rapidly heading back up north instead of dropping down south. It also revs up your metabolism so your body will be burning more calories. What a bonus!

Aim to do three walks each week, and the toning exercises should also be done three times a week. They will only take 10 minutes and can be done from home. It's best to alternate the walking and toning as you need a day's recovery from your toning exercises to let the muscles rest. Whether power pram walking or toning your muscles, always start and finish off doing the stretches as shown on pages 99-101.

Even doing something is better than nothing. Even if you don't do it three times a week, just make time to do something.

How to do the toning exercises

Each exercise has an illustration and description to follow and you will only have one exercise routine to do every other day. The exercises tone lots of muscles in one move - how cool is that? It is what's known as compound exercises, which means they are fab for getting maximum results in minimum time.

Because you are doing these in the comfort of your own home you can wear what you want just as long as it's comfy. Also, because there is no jumping around, you don't need to worry about a sports bra or trainers. Put on your favourite really silly song and do these exercises to your tune - the time goes more quickly and it will only take a few minutes. When it finishes you can have a rest.

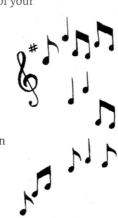

As with the power pram walking, always warm up first, so spend a couple of minutes marching on the spot or up and down the stairs.

Be sure to follow the exercises carefully and put on some music to motivate you. For the floor work, if you don't have a mat, you can always use a towel to protect your back. Always start and finish off with the stretches.

What have I told you about slobbing around in your giant elephant-like trousers? You can wear anything as long as it isn't those huge great 'I-feel-fat trousers'.

How to power pram walk

Walking is one of the most natural and easy forms of exercise that we can do and, let's face it, it's something we do every day without thinking about it. Walking. Simple. Follow some straightforward tips about walking and gain maximum benefit – for a walk's just a walk, and doesn't actually do that much. Why not combine getting a little fresh air for you and your baby, too?

Getting out of the house is so important or you will go nuts!

For your power pram walk, always set off at a slower walk just to ensure that you gently warm up the muscles instead of going from 0 to 60 in 2 seconds as you could cause yourself an injury. Aim for 3 minutes in warm weather and 5 minutes in colder weather for your warm up. To do this, just walk at a decent pace.

Then for the power walking bit, simply walk and push with good posture – stand up straight now please! Make sure that you do not lean forwards to reach the handlebars of the pram. Adjust them if necessary. It is also important that you keep your tummy muscles pulled in and your pelvic floor muscles pulled up (*see* the 'Kegel', don't pee gal on page 33), or the whole thing doesn't work. In fact, it may be an idea to stick a couple of stickers on the pram with just 'tummy' and 'pelvis' written on them as a constant reminder. Walk for as long as is suggested in the exercise programmes on the following pages and then always end with the stretches on pages 99–101.

 Wear a good sports bra, for obvious reasons. Also, wear layers as you will warm up quickly, whatever the weather. Take a bottle of water with you. Not only can you keep properly hydrated (take frequent small sips, especially in the summer), but you will also look

Buggy news

Of course you will be out with the pram not just on days when you are going out for a dedicated pram walk – shopping and general walking around will all add up. Try to walk when you might have previously taken the car.

In a straw poll of recent mothers I have stopped on the streets to ask how they have got back into shape – *all* of them say taking the pram out as often as possible is key to a long and happy life, peace of mind, wealth and new designer clothes everyday (yes, you've caught me out – I made the last bit up).

I've got one of those great three-wheelers. They cost a fortune (thanks Mum!), but they are really neat and go like the clappers. They are really easy to manoeuvre, too. A great investment if you can run to it.

You might also consider a front-loading baby sling – I have seen loads of mum's get fit using these. Try kari-me-baby at www.kari-me.com or www.babybjorn.com.

like you mean business, and can fool anyone at a hundred paces that you are a *serious* exercise fanatic. If you're keen to see the vast distance you've travelled and the number of steps taken – and why not? – get yourself a pedometer, too. Think about getting a fitbug (www.fitbug.co.uk), which is like an up-scale pedometer. It really inspires you to walk further.

Oh yes, and make sure the pram is well cushioned for your baby as you will be travelling a little faster than normal!

 The benefits of walking are endless. It is what is known as low impact, in other words it's less stressful on the joints, unlike other exercises such as running, skipping, or high impact exercise like aerobics and kick boxing, and therefore there is much less chance of injury. Women tend to enjoy walking, so you are more likely to stick to it; it's great for toning your legs, hips, bum, tum and arms. It's also a great fat burner if done correctly.

The key is to be walking at a pace that is fast enough to get you burning fat and toning up. If you take a slow stroll, it won't do you any harm, but neither will you get the effects of an aerobic workout.

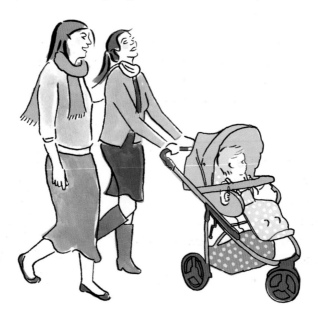

So it's important to walk at the right pace and a good guide for this is to use a scale known as the perceived rate of exertion, also known as the Borg scale.

Blimey, my perceived rate of exertion is massive, carrying the baby up the stairs – she's getting quite big.

Well, here is the perceived rate of exertion scale (known as the PRE) for you to study:

1   **Nothing at all**
2   **Very light**
3   **Light**
4   **Moderate**
5   **Somewhat hard**
6   **Hard**
7   **Very hard**
8   **Very very hard**
9   **Near exhaustion**
10   **Maximal**

As you can see from the chart, a leisurely stroll would have you feeling between a 3 and 4, but to increase your fitness and have a workout it needs to reach a 5 to 5.5.

I prefer to use this chart with clients as opposed to heart rate monitors as a heart rate can be raised by many reasons other than exercises, for example, caffeine, stress, medication and lack of sleep. By using the PRE, though, you know exactly how you are feeling and if you are working hard enough.

It is therefore essential to power pram walk so it feels a level 5, which means you should be feeling slightly out of breath.

Week 1, Day 1

Great! You are out of bed – actually, you have been out of bed twice since 4am. You say to yourself it is not a good day to start healthy living as you are already looking forward to a big glass of cool white wine. Girls! It is only 7am. Look, I never said this was going to be easy, did I? But you do need more sticking power than that. Some days you are going to struggle. Who cares if you cave in once or twice – that is human nature. But don't cave in every day and you will be doing just fine. Keep going.

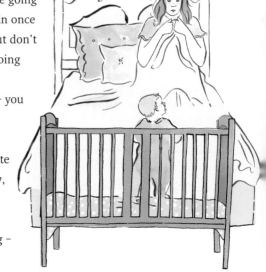

The exercise routine is simple – you spend one day doing this week's exercise routine and then one day doing power pram walking. Alternate this for six days. And then on Day 7, as well as your routine, get out and about for a big long walk with your husband, partner, dog or guinea pig – whoever makes you the happiest.

Today's exercises: The strict butt firm routine

The toning exercises you will be doing this week are all on the floor, so you will need a mat or towel to lie on. They tone your chest, arms, hips, bum, thighs and waist and, by doing them every other day, you will also increase your metabolic rate.

Before doing the exercises, warm up for a couple of minutes as described on page 99 – with nice high legs and as much energy as you can muster. Don't forget to do the stretches, also on pages 99–101, at the end of your session.

I must, I must

What it does: Helps to tone the chest muscles and your triceps, which are the muscles at the back of the upper arms.

What you need: A mat or towel and small hand weights or small full bottles of water.

Hand weights

You can make these easily for yourself by filling two small bottles with water. If you prefer to use manufactured hand weights, then go for 2–3kg (4–6lb). If unsure of how heavy a weight you should start with, it's always best to err on the side of caution. They are available from most good sports shops or you can buy online at www.physicalcompany.co.uk.

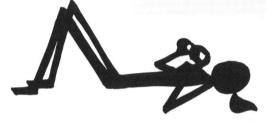

1 Holding onto your weights, lie face up on the mat with knees bent and feet flat on the floor.

2 Hold the weights with an overhand grip and your palms facing your feet. Keep your head and shoulders on the floor.

3 Bend your elbows so that your hands are by your shoulders.

4 Take a deep breath in and then as you breathe out, extend both arms straight up and still in line with the shoulders – avoid locking out the elbows. Hold for a couple of seconds, then slowly lower back to the start position. At all times you must keep your abdominals pulled in to protect your back.

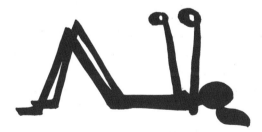

5 Do this 20 times, then rest for a minute and perform a second set.

Nice butt!

What it does: Tones the thighs, hips, butts and abs – what more can you ask for?

What you need: A mat or towel.

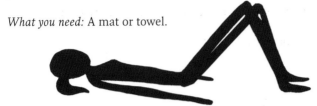

1 Lie face up on the mat with knees bent and feet flat on the floor. Keep your head and shoulders on the floor and put your arms by your sides, with palms facing down.

2 Pressing down with your arms, slowly raise your body until it is straight from your knees to your shoulders. Squeeze your buttocks tight and at all times keep your abdominals pulled in to protect your back.

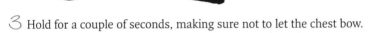

3 Hold for a couple of seconds, making sure not to let the chest bow.

4 Slowly lower yourself back to the start position.

5 Do this 20 times, then rest and perform a second set.

Good times for exercise

* Really early in the morning before your baby has woken up.

* Rest time.

* When you have put your baby to bed.

* If your baby is feeding herself when she is eating – you might get some strange looks (from the baby).

* Just before you go to bed.

Heel taps

What it does: Tones your deepest abdominal muscle, which will help to draw back any separation from your rectus abdominus (the Grand Canyon gap down your middle – your central zipper!) – see page 12.

What you need: A mat or towel.

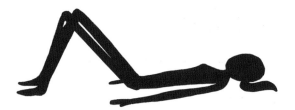

1 Lie face up on the mat with knees bent and feet flat on the floor. Keep your head and shoulders on the floor and put your arms by your sides, with palms facing up.

2 Take a deep breath in and as you breathe out pull your belly button tight towards the spine, then keeping it pulled in, lift one foot off the floor a couple of inches and hold, then slowly lower, ensuring throughout that you have kept your tummy pulled in.

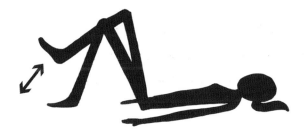

3 Repeat by lifting the other foot. It is important to keep your abdominals pulled in as this is the training effect and also prevents pressure on your back.

4 Alternating legs, aim for 10, then rest and repeat another set.

Today's grub

 Start with a cup of hot water and lemon (wakes up the liver) – yes, yes, I know this is a bit nutritionally worthy, but you really do feel better doing it.

Breakfast: See suggested menus on pages 93–7 for ideas. Actually you don't need to have eggs scrambled – make eggs interesting by having them in any way you like.

Snack: Don't forget to have your snack to keep your blood sugar topped up. You need to be inventive with snacks or they can get really boring.

Lunch: See suggested menu: baked potato with filling. Don't worry if you have forgotten to cook the baked potato. They do take ages to cook, so if you forgot to put it in the oven five hours ago, substitute the potato with some brown rice (which also takes ages to cook, but not as long), quinoa or rye bread. Also, don't worry if you have never heard of some of these weird foods like quinoa (pronounced 'kin-wa' before you make a social gaffe in the health food shop).

Snack: This is the moment your energy might be really flagging – so again, your snack is vital.

Dinner: Make a vegetable stir-fry (be sure not to overcook the vegetables – they should be more steam-fried), smear the pan with some oil and add a sprinkling of water. Then, with the lid on, cook on a highish heat.

A week's menu

These are only suggestions. Use your imagination!
For Brilliant breakfast ideas, see pages 24-7.

Monday

Breakfast

Two scrambled eggs cooked in olive oil or a little organic
unsalted butter, on wholemeal or rye toast; scramble the eggs
with a little spinach or have them with grilled tomatoes.

Mid-morning snack

Sliced pepper (any colour) with hummus or cottage cheese;
mix chilli, spices or pesto with the cottage cheese if you find it
a little bland.

Lunch

Baked potato with grilled or roasted chicken or fish (smoked
mackerel or trout from the supermarket, tinned tuna or salmon
steak) with a salad and steamed or roasted vegetables.

Mid-afternoon snack

An apple or pear or a cup of berries with a small handful of nuts
or seeds.

Dinner

Stir-fry with lots of different coloured vegetables; add some strips
of chicken, turkey, fish or tofu and sprinkle on some seeds just
before serving.

Tuesday

Breakfast

Porridge with nuts, seeds, fresh fruit (chopped, grated or sliced) and yoghurt on top.

Mid-morning snack

Sliced chicken or turkey breast dipped in mustard, pesto or hummus or smoked salmon with lemon.

Lunch

Soup (most supermarkets have a fresh organic range and Covent Garden soups are good, but check for high dairy content) with tuna salad; be creative, add avocado, green beans, peppers, spring onions, apple, chopped fresh herbs, cucumber chunks, cherry tomatoes, radishes, peas and dressing.

Mid-afternoon snack

A piece of fresh fruit and yoghurt (check the label for sugar content).

Dinner

Brown basmati rice (cook enough for lunch tomorrow); add as many of the following as you like: chickpeas, butterbeans, peas, onion, spinach or any vegetables you choose, pieces of grilled/roast chicken or tuna; add herbs, spices and seasonings to taste.

Wednesday

Breakfast

Organic eggs and smoked salmon on wholemeal or wheat-free toast with a sliced tomato.

Mid-morning snack

Rice or oatcakes or rye or gluten-free crackers with cottage cheese or hummus.

Lunch

Brown rice from last night with a piece of grilled/roast chicken, turkey or salmon and a large leafy salad or steamed vegetables.

Mid-afternoon snack

Raw vegetable crudités (cucumber, celery, courgette, pepper, carrot or any other that you fancy) with hummus or avocado dip.

Dinner

Grilled/poached or steamed white fish with lemon, olive oil and herbs with a selection of steamed seasonal vegetables; toss them in oil and/or tamari and add some sesame seeds.

Thursday

Breakfast

Fruit smoothie, adding a handful of porridge oats if you prefer something a little more substantial, but this is very filling on its own; for an extra boost, add a spoonful of 'green food' (spirulina, chlorella, barley greens) or a protein powder.

Mid-morning snack

Boiled egg (try with a little pesto), with some crudités.

Lunch

Soup with a piece of chicken or fish or add tinned tuna to the soup; try adding some chickpeas or butter beans (organic sugar and salt-free varieties are available in tins) and have with a wholemeal roll or wheat-free bread and a little butter.

Mid-afternoon snack

An apple with cottage cheese or yoghurt and a sprinkling of seeds.

Dinner

Grilled lean meat (or fish) on a bed of steamed or roasted vegetables with dressing.

Friday

Breakfast

Porridge with nuts, cinnamon and chopped or grated apple.

Mid-morning snack

A piece of fruit with yoghurt and seeds.

Lunch

Sardines on toast with tomatoes and asparagus.

Mid-afternoon snack

Sliced chicken or turkey breast dipped in mustard, pesto or hummus or smoked salmon with lemon.

Dinner

Casserole with beans and lentils and tofu or chunks of lean meat served with brown basmati rice or quinoa.

Saturday

Breakfast

Two tofu sausages with two poached eggs on wholemeal or wheat-free toast or polenta.

Mid-morning snack

Yoghurt with berries and a handful of nuts.

Lunch

Wheat-free sandwich or wrap with hummus and roasted vegetables with an apple or pear.

Mid-afternoon snack

Sugar-free protein bar with a herbal tea.

Dinner

Chicken or turkey meatballs (or salmon steak) with tomato sauce on a bed of brown basmati rice or quinoa and mixed salad or steamed vegetables, such as spinach, mangetout, peas.

Sunday

Breakfast

Rye toast with smoked salmon and tomatoes and asparagus.

The rest of the day

This is totally up to you, by now you will have a good idea of how to balance your foods, combining protein with carbohydrates. Enjoy, make some time to relax and get an early night to set you up for the week ahead.

Drinks

Remember to drink at least 1.5-2 litres (2½-3½ pints) of bottled or filtered water per day – more if the weather is hot or you are exercising. Try different herb/fruit teas and coffee substitutes as well.

To make salads, vegetables and potatoes a little more interesting:

Try adding extra virgin olive oil, Udo's Choice Ultimate Blend Oil, Omega Essential Balance, pumpkin seed oil, sesame seed oil or make your own dressing by adding a little whole grain mustard, cider or balsamic vinegar or lemon juice and fresh or dried herbs.

Also try adding (not all together, these are just suggestions): grated ginger, orange juice, anchovies, tamari (tastes like soya sauce), honey, paprika, capers and, of course, black pepper.

To make crackers and sandwiches more interesting:

Add avocado, pesto (many different varieties including sun-dried tomato), cottage cheese and hummus to your regular fillings.

Be nice to yourself

Have a lovely bath soak using some delicious bath products by any luxurious make. Really allow yourself to relax, both in body and mind. Take a moment to de-fuzz your legs and other hairy bits and bobs that, like unruly hedges, are getting out of control. The hot water will open the pores of your skin, which will help to give you a much closer shave.

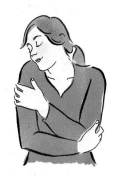

Today's mantra

'I must, I must improve my bust.'

Tick list

Please don't aim to be perfect – just tick off three items that you have done from the list – make one a nutrition thing and one an exercise thing, and one just any old thing.

- I had a really fab breakfast.
- I have staved off any mad cravings.
- I have done The strict butt firm routine.
- I went for a walk.
- I gave myself a little treat of me-time.

Those still breastfeeding?

Make sure you have enough to eat as you guys are burning 500 extra calories. So have a really good breakfast and lunch – add some hemp oil into your baked potato – or you could eat some avocado filled with a dollop of hummus as a starter.

Warm up and stre-t-ch

Warming up

Always make sure the body is warmed up before performing any toning exercises as this will increase your circulation, warm through your muscles and help to prevent injury. Don't be fooled into thinking that just because your toning exercises may only take 5 minutes that you needn't bother with the stretches as this is when an injury can occur.

A warm-up is easy and simple. Literally, just march on the spot for a couple of minutes and towards the end, gently circle through the shoulder joints. Ensure you maintain a good posture with a straight back, tummy pulled in and looking forwards.

Stretching

Whenever you do any exercise, please top and tail them with these stretches. Try to do them in the following order:

Chest stretch

Stand with good posture. Take your arms behind you and lift your shoulders up and back to feel the stretch in the chest.
Hold for 10 seconds.

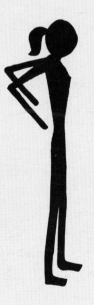

Back of arm stretch

Stand with a strong, firm, straight back (good posture), knees slightly bent, tummy pulled in. Lift one arm up and bend it behind your head, aiming to get your hand between your shoulder blades. Gently support with your other arm. Hold for 10 seconds and then repeat with your other arm.

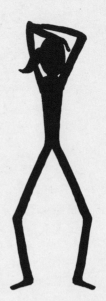

Back stretch

Stand with good posture. Knees are soft and the tummy is pulled in. Take your arms out in front and imagine you are hugging a big beach ball. Feel the stretch through the top of your back. Hold for 10 seconds.

Now for your big muscles and things ...

Calf stretch

Step back with one leg – keep the leg
straight with the heel down but both
feet pointing forwards. Rest your hands
on the bent leg in front. Your head
and back foot should be in a
straight line. Hold for 10
seconds on each leg.

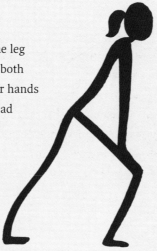

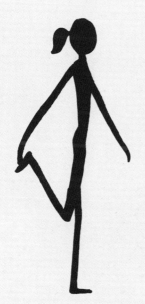

Big fat front of thigh stretch

Standing with a good posture,
bend one leg behind you and
gently hold the foot or sock of the
bent leg. Push your hips forward
to feel the stretch in the front of
the thigh. Keep the supporting leg
slightly bent. Hold for 10 seconds
on each leg.

Week 1, Day 2

Made a total mess-up of yesterday? No problem. Just don't give up that easily. Remember, this is not a diet but a way of life – so in the course of a big long life, straying off the path is of no consequence. So just crack on with today.

Today's exercise: Power pram walking

Get moving and grooving ladies. Put on real exercise clothes (see page 83 for reminders of what to wear and other power pram walking essentials) – remember that you mean business. This is not just an idle walk round the park.

Plan this time, ladies. Don't wait for a 'good' time. Get out (oh, and don't forget the baby) and start by walking for up to 20 minutes. Once you've got more energy, you can look at extending this time.

Today's grub

For suggested menus, see pages 93–7.

Breakfast: Porridge with nuts and seeds and fresh fruit and a dollop of yoghurt. I know porridge is a challenge for some, so why not try muesli as a substitute? I like some of the wheat-free ones, available in health food stores, because they are more likely not to be full of sugar and other nonsense. Although honey is sugar, a tiny drizzle cheers things up, doesn't it? Remember, real porridge – chunky – not the fine, processed versions.

Snacks: Finding good and varied snack ideas is quite difficult on the old imagination. I go for nuts and oatcakes a lot – oatcakes are a good stand-by for stopping you getting *starving* and then going nuts. Remember that if you are starving when eating this way, you are not eating enough food. Keep going with the snacks, though. They are good for keeping the blood sugar topped up.

Lunch: Soup – well, if you can make your own, have a gold star at this point. I like to buy the fresh soups and add my own faves to them to make them chunkier and more filling – you can add fresh broccoli florettes or peas, for example.

Snack: Don't forget your afternoon snack or you will be starving.

Dinner: Brown things, like brown rice and wholemeal pasta take a lot longer to cook, so allow time and check the back of the pack. For breastfeeding, go heavy on the rice and pulses; for the rest of you, go lighter on the rice (a big handful) but eat plenty of pulses.

Trainers (anyone remember the humble plimsole?)
Get a really good pair of training shoes – I get mine from Run and Become (www.runandbecome.com), which specialise in trainers for runners, as well as other bits of gear.

Be nice to yourself

When did you last give yourself a home facial? I *love* the Origins face masks – what a treat (www.origins.co.uk). Get cover from your lovely partner and *lock* the door. It can give someone quite a fright if you look like the ghoul from the deep.

Today's mantra

'When at first you don't succeed, beat yourself up with a stick'. Hang on. That's not how it goes. Be nice to yourself, please.

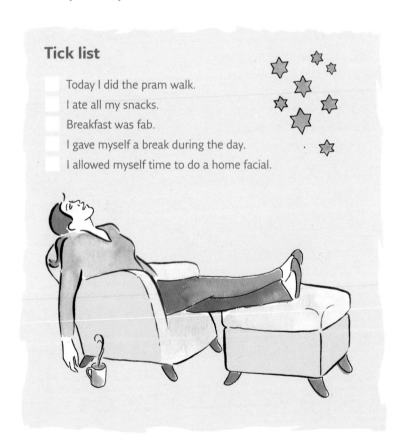

Tick list

- [ ] Today I did the pram walk.
- [ ] I ate all my snacks.
- [ ] Breakfast was fab.
- [ ] I gave myself a break during the day.
- [ ] I allowed myself time to do a home facial.

Mountain climbing

Don't look at the mountain you have to climb with all this fitness/nutrition stuff or it will put you off. Just take one day at a time. You have done really well so far; just keep going and you'll be fine. Don't look at what you haven't done, look at what you have done.

* Think about how it will feel to look brilliant, inside and out. This should encourage you to keep going.
* I know it seems mad, but even tearing out a magazine pic of someone you admire (not for looks but for spirit) can be a positive thing to do. My heroine is Emma Thompson (the British actress), who is smart, intelligent and witty – and lately a glam older mother, too.

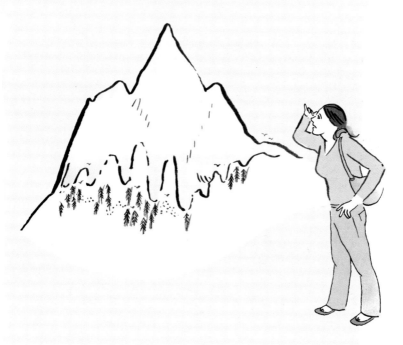

Week 1, Day 3

Rise and shine! Are you ready and raring to go?

Today's exercise: The strict butt firm routine

Get to it! Do some of it, even if you think you are not doing it perfectly. Frankly, don't get in all the gear. Just do it. If you need a reminder for what to do, go back to pages 89–91. Otherwise, here are the pictures, which should act as a reminder.

I must, I must   Nice butt!   Heel taps

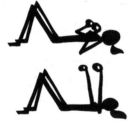
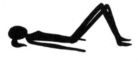
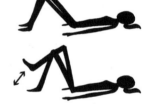

A note about impact

It is essential to avoid any exercise that creates an impact on your body until at least six months from your delivery. Impact is where you are exercising and both feet leave the ground at the same time, like jogging and kick boxing. The reason to avoid these forms of exercise is that you will still have the hormone relaxin floating around your body. This hormone helps loosen the ligaments to allow your baby to come through the pelvis and birth canal more easily. Relaxin isn't just isolated to the pelvis, it affects every single joint, even your little toe. It then remains with you for up to six months after the birth – it is therefore crucial not to over stretch nor make impact moves that could affect the joints.

Fit facts

The benefits of doing your exercises are that they:

* Reduce the risk of heart disease by improving blood circulation throughout the body.
* Keep weight under control.
* Improve blood cholesterol levels.
* Prevent and manage high blood pressure.
* Prevent bone loss.
* Boost energy levels.
* Help manage stress.
* Release tension.
* Improve the ability to fall asleep quickly and sleep well.
* Improve self-image.
* Counter anxiety and depression and increase enthusiasm and optimism.
* Increase muscle strength, which then increases the ability to do other physical activities.
* Provide a way to share an activity with you and your baby by doing MAB exercises (mother and baby) and you can also get local new mums to join in on the walks. Start each week from a different house so that you get to walk varied routes.

Research has shown that people find it easier to stick to a home-based fitness programme, in spite of all the trendy exercise programmes and plush facilities that are now available.

We cannot spot-reduce fat, so if we have flabby thighs, doing thigh exercises alone won't shift the fat, but they will tone the muscle. To get rid of the fat, you need to eat sensibly and put on those trainers and get working aerobically to burn it off.

To get great results you don't have to be pushing yourself to exhaustion for an hour at a time, which many believe and, indeed, puts people off. Instead, it can be just 20 minutes of feeling somewhat challenged. This is great news, as now you know you will stick to it, as opposed to assuming the unrealistic extreme fitness regime.

Today's grub

For suggested menus, see pages 93–7.

Breakfast: More chances to experiment with 100 things to do with an egg today ... the suggestion this morning is eggs with a little bacon (nice organic eggs would be perfect). Remember that bacon is not exactly a health product (all that salt), so go easy on the portion size. Or substitute it for some really good smoked salmon (also salty, so watch the portion size). Wheat-free toast is a lot nicer than it sounds – try anything rye, which you can get at any main supermarket or independent health food shop.

Snacks: Same rule as yesterday – get inventive with your snacking. Remember that if you are eating nuts, go for just a small handful and not the entire packet.

Lunch: I hope you didn't eat all that rice up from yesterday because having it again today for lunch will save you a goodly amount of time waiting for it to cook.

Dinner: Grilled fish with veggies – I get packets of fresh fish and freeze them, then you can just take them out of the freezer as you require. Tamari is a wheat-free soya sauce from Japan; you should be able to get it from any health food shop.

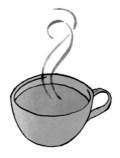

Be nice to yourself

Have a square of Green & Black's dark organic chocolate and really enjoy it!

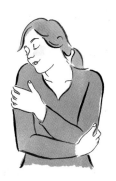

Today's mantra
'A journey of a thousand steps starts with a toned butt.'

Spoil yourself!
I hope you have bought yourself some nice kit to do the exercise stuff in – it makes you feel so much better than a huge baggy T-shirt. I often see girls these days (sound like my mum) in really tight gear when they are really quite large. I have to hand it to them – at least they are out there, even if it is all a little in your face. So go on, flaunt it. Try Sweaty Betty for really nice stuff (www.sweatybetty.com).

Tick list

☐ I ate breakfast.
☐ I did the butt stuff exercises.
☐ I didn't eat all the rice from yesterday and had some left over for today (score 4 extra points).
☐ I exercised in nice gear – no giant T-shirt/elephant trousers for me.
☐ By the end of the day I was still on course.

Week 1, Day 4

I bet that by now you have managed to score millions of points on your tick lists. I'm very proud of you – not that you need that from me. Remember – look at what you are managing to do, not what you are not managing to do. So, a sneaky bit of chocolate? Don't worry. The whole bar? Do better tomorrow.

Today's exercise: Power pram walking

If you haven't so far managed to incorporate your pram walking into daily life, then no excuse – get out now. There is never a good time to get out of the house – there is always just one more thing to do – so don't wait for all the planets to be aligned, just do it.

Today's grub

For suggested menus, see pages 93–7.

Breakfast: Slurp on a smoothie. If you want to feel fuller, then add a little protein powder (Solgar do one called Whey to Go) and some essential fatty acids (good fats). Udo's oil would be fine. Do put in a handful of oats as this will chunk it out. It should be a thickish drink by the time you have finished with it, not something you could glug down in one.

Snack: Choose some yummy snack suggestions today.

Lunch: Combine a tin of organic (if possible) chickpeas with chopped tomatoes, chopped cucumber, a bit of tuna, coriander and some feta cheese to cheer it up. Add a drizzle of oil and a squeeze of lemon. You could also use some freshly cooked lentils.

Dinner: Adding herbs and spices really perks up food – ginger or coriander can change the nature of a meal into a more oriental offering, for example. See what you think.

Be nice to yourself

Get your mum (or other willing victim) to come round and baby-sit and either: a) go out and get your nails done or b) if you have a steady hand and patience, do it yourself.

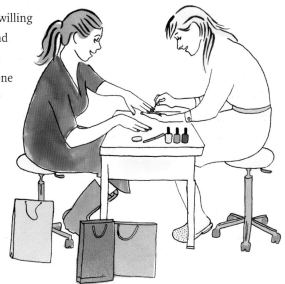

Today's mantra
'**Don't suffer to be beautiful – get someone else in to do my beauty treatments for me.**'

What's under there?

Work out where and what you have to do today and incorporate your pram walk so you are not making a special trip. It is permitted to go out in your exercise gear as long as you have invested in decent clothes.

While you are at it, make sure you have nice underwear on, too – not too many cycles in the washing machine please so that that your knickers are a shade of grey. Just because you are a mummy doesn't mean that everything has to go to pot.

Tick list

- I treated myself today.
- I had a good breakfast (score 5 extra points).
- I did my pram walk today.
- I sat down once today.
- I remembered to eat my snacks.

Week 1, Day 5

It's nearly the weekend – not that this means anything in babyland where there's never a day off. But, smile and the world smiles with you.

Today's exercise: The strict butt firm routine

 Yes, folks, you get the picture. Need a reminder? Go back to pages 89–91; otherwise, here are those pictures.

| I must, I must | Nice butt! | Heel taps |

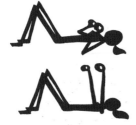 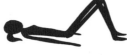 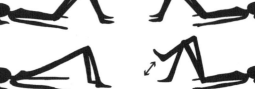

Today's grub

 For suggested menus, see pages 93–7.

Breakfast: Porridge with a little cinnamon spices it up (excuse the pun) – and this flavoursome spice helps balance your blood sugar, too. Remember that if you don't like porridge to choose an alternative, like muesli – you don't have to follow all this to the letter. Porridge isn't such a schlep to cook as you might think – the trick is to cook it on a slow heat topping up with water every so often (see also page 25).

Snacks: The snacks today should be as appetising as your meals – so have fun. Try avocado dips, tapenades (olive pastes), hummus or a little cottage cheese.

Lunch: OK, sardines are not everyone's idea of a good time – if you hate the thought of opening a smelly tin of the blighters, then why not have a salad Niçoise or a smoked mackerel fillet? Or get up early and catch your own sardines and grill them over an open fire – now wouldn't that be lovely?

Dinner: Casserole with beans, lentils and chickpeas – really easy. Stir-fry some onions, celery, peppers and garlic in a heavy pan, add two tins of tomatoes and a tin of chickpeas (if this doesn't feel thick enough for you, add another half tin). If not breastfeeding, add a bit of red chilli (the real ones, deseeded). On serving (with brown rice, of course), add masses of coriander.

Be nice to yourself

Lock yourself in the bathroom (again! Your partner is going to think you have a secret lover – chance would be a fine thing) and exfoliate. Give yourself a good old scrub.

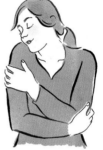

Today's mantra

'OMMMMM OMMMM OMMMM.' Take a deep breath and try saying this out loud – those Buddhists know a thing or two about calming the mind.

Tick list

I have been nice to myself today and given myself a treat.
I have done Nice butt!
I got out of the house today.
I have had breakfast.
I have smiled. (If laughed, too, you get 12 extra points.)

Week 1, Day 6

Good stuff – Day 6 already and, guess what, don't worry if the whole thing has turned to filth already – just keep going with some of it. If you have just been doing the pram walking bit, *that is fine* and better than nothing. When you are ready, do the toning bits, too. Who knows? You might like the soft squidgy bits.

Today's exercise: Power pram walking

Head down the park/road at a really fast pace – got the pram and the baby? Great start.

Today's grub

For suggested menus, see pages 93–7.

Breakfast: Look, just try a tofu sausage and see how you get on before you turn your hooter up at this idea. But if you can't face it, then a Spanish omelette would be a fab alternative – just chuck in anything you fancy to bulk it up (food obviously). If this day happens to fall on a Saturday, I am generalising horribly, but blokes tend not to like things like tofu, so to get your loved one on side, the Spanish omelette might be better all round.

Snacks: Remember that snacks are not like a whole other meal – if you cup your palm, the snack should fit in the dent. Don't try to pile them up like a Scooby snack.

Lunch: Try a rye bread sandwich – avocado or hummus with watercress. Delicious.

Dinner: Try red quinoa instead of the normal quinoa – do add a stock cube for flavouring (makes it just about 100 times nicer) and you can also cheer things up by adding herbs at the last minute – mint sprigs, for example.

Be nice to yourself

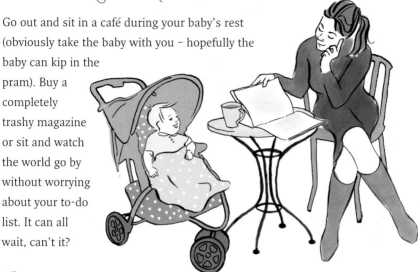

Go out and sit in a café during your baby's rest (obviously take the baby with you – hopefully the baby can kip in the pram). Buy a completely trashy magazine or sit and watch the world go by without worrying about your to-do list. It can all wait, can't it?

Today's mantra

You can sing this, taken from Monty Python's Life of Brian: 'Always look on the bright side of life, der dum, der dum, der der der der der dum.' If you don't know what I am talking about, get the film out (www.lovefilm.com) – a rare treat.

When you are out with the pram don't multitask but focus on all the great things you have in your life ... a beautiful baby, a home, a loving partner. It is easy to look on the dark side of life and before too long sink into a pit of despair.

Tick list

- I got out to a really good film and had a good old blub.
- I have done my pram walking.
- I called three girlfriends and had a gossip in rest hour.
- I have had my breakfast.
- I have been nice to my partner today.

Week 1, Day 7

OK ladies – now you may think that Day 7 should be a day of rest. Oh, how *wrong* can you be. But because I'm feeling nice you can either do The strict butt firm routine or take a long walk with your partner or anyone else who will join you. Oh yes, no skiving off now. I will let you off to go to church and *that* is it.

Today's exercise: The strict butt firm routine

 Up and at 'em – you've done a whole week. Great stuff!

I must, I must   Nice butt!   Heel taps

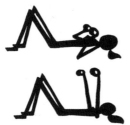 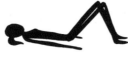 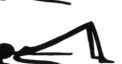 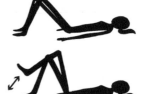

Today's grub

 For suggested menus, see pages 93-7.

Breakfast: If this day does happen to be a Sunday, then the suggested breakfast on page 97 is a great start to the day, especially if you are going to have a heavier roast lunch.

Lunch: If you do plan to have a family meal today, remember there are always ways of doing better – so don't eat spuds and parsnips (white and fluffy) and really up the veg. Loads of gravy probably isn't a health product. If pudding is fruit, then so much the better.

Dinner: If you have had a roast at lunch, try to think of dinner as a lighter snack rather than another meal – a soup and some rye toast would be fine. I just had a fabulous Moroccan chickpea soup; it was filling and delicious, too. I obviously made it myself this morning from my own chickpeas ... I don't think so. Some of the organic soups you can buy are fine – go with that and make life easier for yourself.

Be nice to yourself

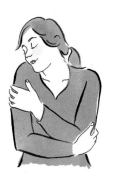

Get your partner to take over the kids for the morning – and instead of making the house perfect and getting your chores done, go and do grown up things – like going to an art exhibition or whatever floats your boat. Don't feel guilty.

Today's mantra
'Screw it, let's do it!', as Richard Branson would say – get out there and enjoy.

A guilt trip is not a vacation

Don't feel guilty about anything – well, unless you have been shoplifting (obviously). Guilt is a little prompt from the subconscious mind to make us change our behaviour and to be a good girl – but who has defined what a good girl is? Our parents? Our teachers? When we are adults this definition of good and bad might be totally out of line with who we are now. So as soon as you hear yourself say 'should', you know that is a guilt word. Quit the 'should' words!

Tick list

- I have decided not to feel guilty about things (200 points).
- I have done my pram walking.
- I have lolled in a deep bath with luscious potions.
- I have had breakfast.
- I have eaten two snacks to keep my blood sugar propped up.

Week 2

Great stuff everyone! You got through week one. You must be feeling better already. Sometimes you can even start feeling better after one day. And don't worry if you weren't perfect – I know I have said that before but so what if the odd cream bun crept in? This is not a diet.

And without sounding like a boring old soul, the exercise bit really does work, so even if you do half of what Lucy is suggesting you will be a new woman before you know it. If you hate the toning exercises, at least make sure you do the pram walking instead – don't force yourself to do something you really don't like.

Anyway ... this week. Since you now know the format, I am going to give you some guidelines for the week without actually guiding you through every day. In that way, as you know your own preferences and timetables, you will be able to fit the 'new way' around your baby and your life.

If you had any challenges or problems with last week, it is worth just having a little think about what worked and what didn't work, so that you can sort it out now and begin afresh.

* Having trouble getting the food in? Consider deliveries.
* Having trouble making time? Look at your priorities – do you really want to change? Perhaps get your mum to come round so that you can grab some time to get out.

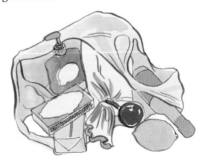

* Are you just too knackered and finding that taking on a whole change of routine is all too much? If so, you might want to abandon ship and come back to this nutrition and health stuff later. You have a huge excuse to be tired, just don't let it stop you doing stuff forever.
* Are you trying to be too much of a perfectionist? A perfect wife, mum and now super-duper fitness guru. Just take every day as it comes and promise yourself no more than that. Just keep taking the steps and you will get there. If everything turns to filth – just concentrate on:
    - Focusing on breakfast.
    - Focusing on pram walking.

So, ready for Week 2?

This week's exercises: The bright new dawn routine

As for Week 1, do your new routine every other day, alternating with the pram power walking. This week's routine is called The bright new dawn routine because this is almost the beginning of the Bright New Dawn of getting back into shape.

* Remember to warm up.
* Remember to stretch both before and after the routine.

Toning exercises really do increase your metabolic rate – so you can have more cream buns.

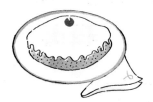

No! No! No! That's not how it goes.

Drawing the curtains

What it does: This will help to tone the pectorals major, which is the muscle that supports the bust, and also tone your triceps at the back of your upper arms.

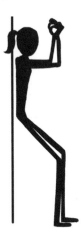

What you need: Small hand weights or small full bottles of water and a wall.

1 Holding onto your weights, stand by a wall with your feet about 30cm (12in) in front, with knees slightly bent and the feet a hip-width distance apart. Keep the rest of your body pressed into the wall.

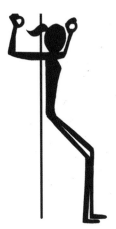

2 Lift your arms out to the side to shoulder height with your body, still in contact with the wall and palms facing forwards. Raise your arms at the elbows so that your arms form an L-shape and the elbows are still in line with the shoulders.

3 Take a deep breath in and then as you breathe out bring both the arms together so that your forearms meet in the middle, still keeping them at shoulder height. Breathe in and return to the start position. To get your abdominals working on this one make sure you keep your belly button pulled tight to the spine and be sure not to let your back arch.

4 Aim to do this 20 times, then rest for a minute and perform a second set.

Your wee one

Depending on the age of your little one – either put her in the highchair with some toys or small ones can go in their bouncer and watch (and have a jolly good laugh). Bigger toddlers can join in. I know this sounds remarkably unhelpful but my lovely 20-month bundle of joy likes to copy me doing my exercises – actually it is really funny. Well, she likes to have a laugh.

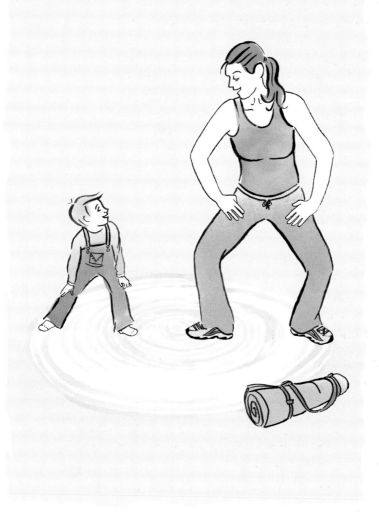

Puppet on a string

What it does: Works deep into your core muscles, helping to reduce the separation. Even though you are lifting the leg, don't be fooled into thinking this is a leg exercise, as this totally works your abs and, by lifting the leg, ups the resistance for the tummy.

What you need: Yourself and a wall.

1 Stand by a wall with your feet about 30cm (12in) in front, with knees slightly bent and feet a hip width distance apart. Stand with good posture. Let your arms hang down by your side, with the palms facing the wall.

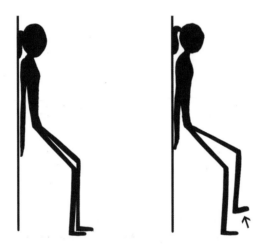

2 Take a deep breath in and as you breathe out pull your navel in towards your spine at the same time as gently lifting one foot off the floor. Hold for a second, still keeping your tummy pulled in, then lower your leg and release the abdominals. At all times you must keep your abdominals pulled in to protect your back as you lift your leg.

3 Repeat using the opposite leg and remember to breathe out as you pull your tummy in.

4 Aim for 20 alternating the legs, then rest and repeat another set.

Up and down

What it does: Tones your buttocks, thighs and abs, plus this is a great way of increasing your metabolic rate.

What you need: Yourself and a wall.

1 Standing against the wall, with feet a hip width distance apart and several inches in front of you, slowly bend your knees so you are sliding down the wall.

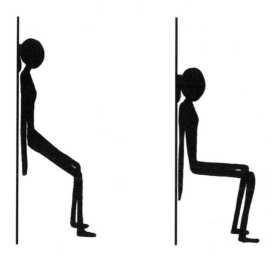

2 Slide down until your thighs are approximately in line with the floor, but make sure your knees don't shoot over the line of your toes.

3 Slowly push with your legs to the return position. Breathe out as you slide down and breathe in on the way up. Remember to keep your tummy pulled in.

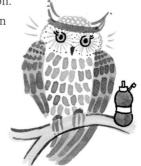

4 Aim for 20, then rest and repeat another set.

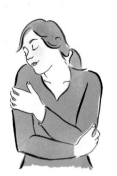

Be nice to yourself

What about arranging a trip to go out to lunch with a friend? Is the baby still young enough to take with you without causing too many problems? Or could a friend come round to yours for lunch during rest time at home?

There are also a couple of musts for this week:

You MUST have breakfast

Don't get uninspired for breakfast – remember to try and eat protein where you can.

* What about rye toast with cashew nut butter topped with tomatoes and coriander?
* What about muesli with rice milk and berries, a sprig of mint and Greek yoghurt?
* What about kedgeree (your mum must have a recipe)?
* What about sardines on toast?
* What about asparagus and poached egg/scrambled egg with good smoked salmon?
* What about cold cooked salmon?
* Or how about healthy pancakes with fillings such as tomatoes and goat's cheese with rocket (replace the wheat flour with buckwheat flour to ring the changes).

You might be groaning and thinking that you just don't have time for all this. Well, you do have time. You just might not be prioritising it right now. You don't have time not to have time – because breakfast will *save you*. I am seriously thinking of retiring and putting a large notice on the clinic door. It would read:

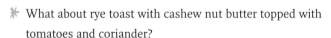

'BREAKFAST'
Kate Cook has now retired
and gone to live on a desert island.

You MUST do your pram walking

I had quite an overweight lady in my clinic the other day, but we identified that she could really make a difference with some exercise in her life so she elected to walk the dog for an hour. But the walking she was doing was the, 'Hello clouds, hello pretty flowers' type of walking and, of course, it was making not a jot of difference, even if the dog was happy. You need to keep the pace up ladies. No ambling. There is always a time and a place for ambling certainly, but not if you want to get fit.

Dinner

I find that early suppers work best so either go out once your partner is back or cook something really easy at home. Tonight we have grilled organic salmon with salad followed by raspberries and strawberries and vanilla yoghurt. Now how easy and yummy is that?

Tick list

I am still doing the toning exercises – score 100 points.
I gave myself a treat.
I ate breakfast.
I did my pram walking.
I was nice to my partner.
I didn't burst into tears with all those late nights with the baby teething.
Add lots of other brilliant things
that I have done each day.

Week 3

This week is where you might start to see a real difference – if you are skim reading through the book, have faith. You just reached Week 3 ... you can do it, I know you can. You can expect to feel the trousers feeling just a little less sprayed on and you may also experience a bit of let up in the tiredness department. Furthermore, your skin could start to look a little more glowing. Great work!

How were your potential problems and challenges last week? What did you find easy and what did you find difficult? What would you do differently? Try to look at what you did right rather than what you did wrong, though. Humans are funny creatures – we are so busy bashing ourselves up for the bits we didn't do rather than the bits we did perfectly well. I suppose this strategy did get our ancestors off their butts and out of the cave – if they had been happy with the des res cave arrangement, well, life would have been very different indeed. However, this needing everything to be perfect sometimes makes us want to give up. 'Stuff it,' you cry, 'why do I even bother? This making an effort isn't working – look at how fat my stomach still is.' We feel that we are not somehow doing enough, but even doing a little is going to have an impact. Even if you just focused on the main items last week – the breakfast thing and pram walking – then that is *good*.

Getting used to a new routine and accepting change is very rarely a lightning strike, with all the old habits magically turning into worthy new habits. Change evolves and sometimes that takes time.

This week's exercises: The big boys routine

This week's adventure is called The big boys routine simply because it works the big muscle groups, which means you'll also be burning off extra calories.

* Do them every other day with the pram walking in between.
* Don't forget to warm up.
* Don't forget to stretch (see pages 99–101).

Superwoman wonder wall

What it does: It might not seem like it, but with this one you are holding up the wall all by yourself. What strength! It is great for toning your chest, lifting up the bust, tightening the back of the upper arms and for work on the tummy.

What you need: Yourself and a wall.

1 Facing a sturdy wall, stand three steps away from it. Place your palms flat on the wall and slightly wider than shoulder width distance apart at chest level. Your body should be in a straight line from head to toe.

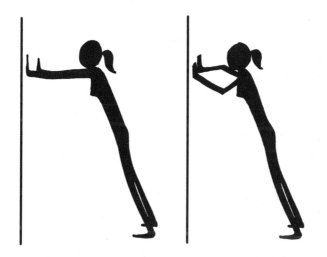

2 Keeping your arms a shoulder width apart and tummy pulled in, lower yourself towards the wall by bending your elbows out to the sides.

3 When your arms are at a right angle, pause and straighten to repeat. At all times you must keep your abdominals pulled in to protect your back.

4 Aim for 15, then rest and repeat another set.

Tummy tightener

What it does: Says what it does on the tin. This is one of the most basic abdominal exercises, but one of the most important to help repair that separation. I am a great advocator for tummy exercises – go for quality as opposed to quantity.

What you need: A mat or towel.

1 Lie face up on the mat with knees bent and feet flat on the floor. Place your hands by your ears.

2 Breathing out, lift your head slightly, curling your shoulders forwards as you do. Keep your back on the floor and, most importantly, pull your belly button tight to your spine. Hold for a second then slowly lower, breathing in as you do.

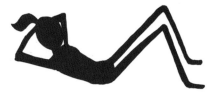

3 Perform these very slowly and focus on feeling this working in your tummy muscles. Don't try to lift too high and if you feel any tension in your neck, stop and rest for several seconds then start again.

4 Aim for 10, then rest and repeat another set.

Curtsey to the queen

What it does: This is a great exercise for the lower body as it tones up your buttocks, quads (the big thigh muscles) and hamstrings as well as working your core muscles.

1 Stand straight in a split stance, with your feet about a metre (yard) apart and knees softly bent.

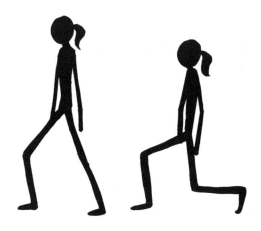

2 Bend both knees to about 90-degree angles, being sure to keep the upper body straight. Then slowly push through the front heel to come back to the start position, making sure you don't lock the knees out as you straighten up.

3 Aim to do this 20 times, then rest for a minute and perform a second set.

Ear, ear

I know this sounds, well, weird, but to pick up your energy, try pinching your ears. Work down your ears to the lobe, pinching firmly between the finger and thumb. Origins (www.origins.co.uk) do a sensory therapy 'Peace of Mind' peppermint oil, which is truly fab. You rub it in – this makes your ears hot, but it is all a lot better than it sounds. Have a go for instant refreshing calm.

Be nice to yourself

 Go and get yourself a nice outfit – or even just a pretty top. Now, I would hate to encourage you to be extravagant, but these days some of the cheaper shops are actually better than the designer megabucks places anyway. Go with a friend and let her pick you out something that perhaps you would never normally wear – whether it's a different style or a bold colour.

Then there are this week's two musts:

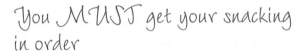

You MUST get your snacking in order

At first snacking seems to be a bit counter intuitive – we are so used to the slap on the wrist for picking at food. Well, snacking is very different to picking. Picking is about grazing on all the 'wrong' stuff (right and wrong are not part of our vocabulary). A bit of cheese straight from the fridge and a nibble of a chocolate biscuit that has been hanging around, or just finishing up the dregs of your daughter's spaghetti and tomato sauce – well, it does seem such a shame to let it go to waste, doesn't it?

Ideally, a snack should have a bit of protein in it to keep your blood sugar stable. The aim of snacking is to keep your energy topped up so that you are not so starving hungry that your eyes are bigger than your stomach and you start making poor choices by turning in to some manic gobbling *monster*. Your day could therefore go:

7am Breakfast

10.30am Snack

1pm Lunch

4pm Snack

7.30pm Dinner

For some continued snack inspiration, try:

❋ Yoghurt with a pinch of cinnamon.

❋ Hummus on oatcake with cucumber.

❋ A little cottage cheese on a rye cracker with chopped chives.

❋ You can always grab some nuts and seeds but just watch how much you are eating – only give yourself a small handful to take the edge off your hunger.

You MUST try to do some of the toning exercises this week

Even if you just chose to do the ones in the preparation section (the Super Seven) and decided that you wouldn't use the specific exercises that have been laid out for you every week, now is the time to reverse that decision. Please, please, please try some of them. Don't get intimidated into thinking of the whole picture. Do something. Anything will do.

Tick list

I went out and had a makeover.

I did some of the exercises.

I had breakfast.

I actually stopped and had lunch rather than having a crispbread (this earns you 15 extra points).

I went out and did my pram walking.

Week 4

Well done, folks. Can you believe we are up to Week 4 already, and hasn't it been a mega-packed fun trip full of fabulous frolics? Now look here, Lucy and I have been doing our best. And for an added bonus, your energy really should be much revived by now. Well, revved up might be a tad strong, but well done for getting to grips with all this - it's a great achievement with all the other things you are doing in your life.

The usual question, what were your trials, tribulations and challenges last week? Don't worry if the whole thing has descended into chaos, just concentrate on what you are doing well - and don't give up just because you are not doing 1,000 pelvic floors a minute.

Don't forget to ask for help. Us women are useless at asking for what we need - our partners, friends and family really want this to be a success for us, so rope them in to give you a hand with childcare arrangements or time where you can get out of the house and be a grown-up somewhere.

This week's exercises: The super heroes routine

You should really start to be noticing a difference now as you will be feeling more toned, fitter and stronger. This week's exercises are called The super heroes routine because that's what you are. The exercises focus on toning the arms, still working on the abdominal repair and a great exercise for the lower body that tones hips, thighs legs, butt *and* abdominals all in one move.

* Do them every other day with the pram walking in between.
* Don't forget to warm up.
* Don't forget to stretch (see pages 99–101).

Wonder Woman waist

What it does: Now there's something to aim for! As for last week, this is exactly the same as Tummy tightener, but you are going to add an extra lift to work your abs a little harder.

What you need: A mat or towel.

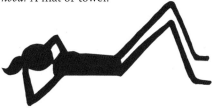

1 Lie face up on the mat with your knees bent and feet flat on the floor. Place your hands by your ears.

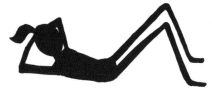

2 Breathing out, lift your head slightly, curling your shoulders forwards as you do. Keep your back on the floor and, most importantly, pull your belly button tight to your spine. Hold for a second then lift an inch higher still, keeping your tummy pulled in.

3 Perform these very slowly and focus on feeling this working in your tummy muscles. At all times you must keep your abdominals pulled in to protect your back.

4 Aim for 10, then rest and repeat another set.

First sign of madness – a super-tidy home

I know it is really tempting to get on with essential house tidying when the baby is sleeping, but when he is kipping grab your moment to do the exercises instead – you might not get a second chance.

Ballet butt

What it does: Tones your inner and outer thighs, buttocks, hips and abs, plus this is a great way of increasing your metabolic rate.

1 Stand with your feet wider than a hip width apart and have your toes out at a 45-degree angle. Keep your upper body in good posture with shoulders pulled back and abs in tight.

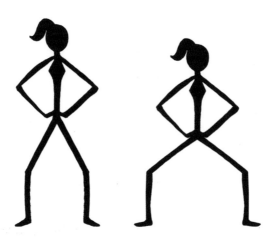

2 Slowly bend through the knees while keeping your upper body straight. Make sure that your knees don't go over the line of your toes.

3 Hold for a second at the lowest level, then slowly return to the start position.

4 Aim for 20, then rest and repeat another set.

Yes, miss! Yes, miss!

What it does: This exercise helps to tone the triceps, which are the muscles at the back of the upper arms. Combine this exercise with walking and you will tone to perfection.

What you need: A chair and small hand weights or small full bottles of water.

1 Holding one hand holding a weight, sit on a chair, with good posture and your abdominals pulled in.

2 Extend the hand holding the weight directly up in the air and then, with the other hand, support the arm. Now simply bend the extended arm with the weight at the elbow.

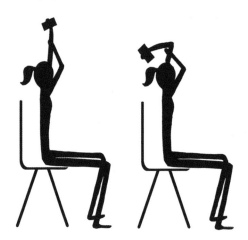

3 Slowly straighten the arm, using the other arm just to help keep the elbow in line with the shoulder.

4 Aim to repeat 15 times, then swap arms, rest for a minute and perform a second set.

There are no shortcuts to any place worth going!
I know that at first exercise seems like it will make sod all difference, so why do it? But over time I promise you that it is really the key to getting back your energy, never mind your body. But the change is sometimes slow and you will not notice anything straightaway – so vow to just get on with it and do it – and don't *look* for the result.

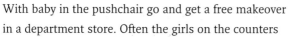

Be nice to yourself

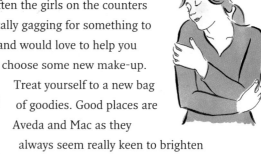

With baby in the pushchair go and get a free makeover in a department store. Often the girls on the counters are totally gagging for something to do and would love to help you choose some new make-up. Treat yourself to a new bag of goodies. Good places are Aveda and Mac as they always seem really keen to brighten up your day.

You MUST look at portion sizes

... unless you are still breastfeeding, as eating naturally healthy food will mean that you are dropping weight any way and, as you know, breastfeeding makes you hungry enough to eat a huge horse. Don't attempt to adjust your portion sizes downward if you are eating good, fresh, natural food. Of course, if you are eating junk food or huge elephant-sized portions then we might be having a different discussion.

For the rest of you, (boring, boring, boring, I know) you can't just eat mega portions and expect it not to have an effect on your weight. It is just the way of the world.

With a little planning

Make loads of chunky soups and freeze them in individual portion-sized plastic containers. When you need a lunch, get one of the containers out of the freezer and serve with some salad (leaves, chickpeas, peppers, cucumber, tomatoes) and some crispbread such as the Spelt Dr Karg's, the unfeasibly great crispbread from Germany. What an instant fab lunch. Now that's what I call convenience.

* If you cup your hands slightly, your portion size should be no more than you can fit into your outstretched hands.
* You should be having about 40 per cent protein and 60 per cent veg (complex carbohydrates – that is, food with loads of fibre content).
* Of that 60 per cent, around 20 per cent could be stuff like brown rice, sweet potatoes or millet – or the more starchy carbohydrates (*see* page 62 to remind yourself of what this means).

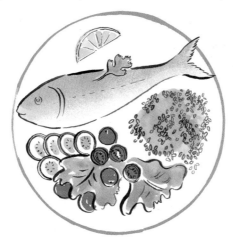

You MUST eat real food

This, after all, is Rule 5 of our guidelines on page 48. I know it is a hassle to prepare food, but there is no such thing (really) as healthy convenience food, whatever they tell you. Of course, there will be times when the knackered-you wins and before you know it your fingers are on the dial to your local takeaway. If you do succumb, make it better by:

* Cooking your own brown rice.
* Cooking your own veg.
* Doing away with the sauces or choosing the stuff on the menu without the sauces.
* Chucking away the free naan bread.
* Drinking water instead of alcohol.

Keeping up your exercising

Power walking

Why not find a local charity walk race? There are so many, like the Race for Life, the distance of which is 5km (3 miles). You will have a goal to work towards and to make it even more fun, get some girlfriends to do it with you. This will get you super fit and gives you a massive feeling of self-achievement when you have participated.

Swimming

This is great as there is no stress on the joints and so no impact; also it's fun.

Circuits at home

From Week 5 you could choose seven different exercises and draw them up on your own circuit cards. Turn your front room into your own gym, put on some motivating music and do one minute on each exercise. For an extra good workout, do the circuit twice, and for the super fit, repeat the circuit three times.

Find something fun

In addition to your toning exercises, take up something fun like line dancing or salsa. Even better, these are low impact so gentle on the joints.

At the gym

If you are a gym member, always tell the instructors so they can help you with a programme. The best bits of equipment for you would be the recumbent bike as opposed to the upright bike as your spine is fully supported. The treadmill is also good, but make sure you are only walking and be aware to keep your tummy pulled in and walk with good posture. If you use steppers and cross trainers, don't lock out your joints, work in a smaller range of movement and avoid excessive pelvic movement.

If you are used to training in the gym and use weights, use the weight machines rather than free weights and set them to a smaller range of movement. Lift lighter weights, keep those tummy muscles pulled in and keep the exercises very slow and controlled.

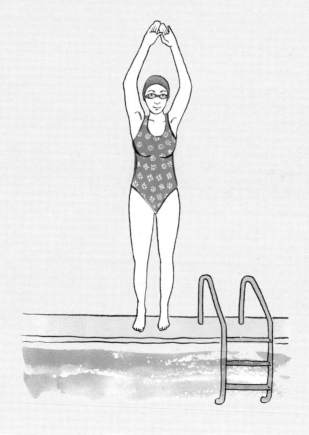

Week 5

You are into your second month already. Fabulous stuff. As you have got this far, I am going to start to let go of your hand just a little bit more. Sniff, Sniff. I'll miss you.

This week's exercises: Kissing your baby routine — MMMWAAA!

I have designed the exercises so you can do them with your baby, the exercises look at toning the chest, arms, lifting your bottom and toning deep into your abdominals.

Kiss the baby press up

What it does: Tones the chest, back of the upper arms and abdominals. You must keep the tummy pulled in throughout this exercise.

What you need: A mat or towel and your baby (or substitute).

1 Kneel on the mat on all fours, with knees under hips and hands under shoulders. Fingers facing forwards.

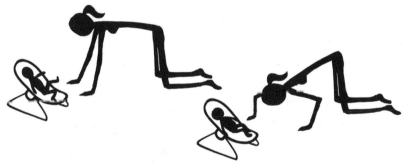

2 Pulling your navel to your spine, at the same time bend your elbows to lower your upper body towards the floor as if you are going to kiss your baby. Then slowly push back up, being sure not to lock out your elbows when your arms are straight.

3 Aim for 20 of these, rest and repeat another set.

Kiss your baby and leg lift

What it does: This is great for toning the buttocks and hamstrings and working the abdominals at the same time. Keep your abdominals pulled in, not only to tone them but also to protect your back.

What you need: A mat or towel and your baby (or substitute).

1 Kneel on the mat on elbows and knees, with elbows under shoulders and forearms facing forwards. Draw your navel to the spine and extend one leg behind with foot flexed and toes resting on the floor. Have your baby by your arms so you can maintain eye contact.

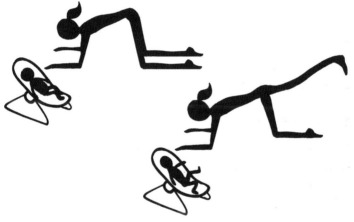

2 Take a deep breath in and as you breathe out, pull in your tummy muscles and slowly raise the extended leg to hip level, squeezing tight into the buttock muscle. Hold for one second then slowly lower with control.

3 Aim for 15 each leg, rest and repeat another set.

Kiss your baby, Supermum

What it does: This is a challenging exercise as you encourage the balance of your whole body through the contraction of your deep abdominal muscles. This is an abdominal exercise so it is essential to keep the belly button pulled in tight.

What you need: A mat or towel and your baby (or substitute).

1 Kneeling on all fours on the mat with your baby in front of you, place your wrists under your shoulders and knees under your hips. Make sure your spine is straight and contract your abdominals.

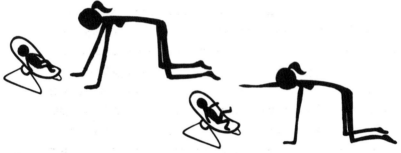

2 Slowly stretch one arm directly in front so it is in line with your torso and aim to hold for 4 seconds keeping your abdominals tight at the same time. Then slowly lower the arm back down to the start position. Alternate with your arms, maintaining eye contact with your baby while you perform the exercise.

3 Aim for 12 repeats, alternating the arms. Rest and repeat another set.

 If you have come to this later and your baby is moving around the room uncontrollably, either get granny in to baby-sit or do the exercises in rest hour using a teddy as a replacement for your baby!

Be nice to yourself

Get some books on CD as they are great to listen to while doing things around the house. If you can handle it, try brushing up on some English Lit with a Jane Austen CD. At least you'll be perking up the grey matter.

You MUST go out

Book a baby-sitter now.

You MUST think about your nutrition

I am sure that by now you have got the hang of the nutritional stuff. If you are struggling, well, you know not to bash yourself up as that is definitely against the rules. Instead of wasting energy hitting yourself on the head with a hairbrush and wondering why you could have been so weak willed as to pile into the cream buns, look at the reasons. Not the excuses, but the reasons.

If you find yourself comfort eating – reaching for the biscuits when you are definitely not hungry – perhaps there is another psychological reason why you are still not with the programme. The other day I had a lady in the clinic whose mum ran dieters clubs and took her to her first session (weigh-ins and the lot) aged six. She, of course, has been on a constant diet since she was knee-high to a grasshopper. Even I can work out that this could be a cause of her constant struggle with her weight. Luckily she knows this, too, and is seeing a hypnotherapist about it.

Another reason for reaching for the biscuit tin is just being plain knackered. Try to have acceptable snacks for the super tired moments – nuts, seeds and fruit. Also consider whether you are dehydrated (especially if you are breastfeeding).

You MUST remember your partner

Don't forget your partner in the whirl of baby stuff. Don't forget to kiss him every day – he is not just the relief shift. This oils the cogs of your relationship and makes for a more harmonious home.

Tick list

I had breakfast.
I kissed my partner and told him I loved him.
I involved my baby in some of the exercises I am doing.
I had a laugh (score 35 extra points).
I booked a baby-sitter and went out (*ping!* Score 100 points).

Week 6

I am very proud of you all – not that you need any more gold stars from me.

How are you doing on lunch? Lunch is the most difficult meal to fit in as it is a bore to only prepare something for one. However, if you are weaning, then it is a really good discipline to cook for you both. I don't believe in giving babies special food, so depending where you are on the weaning cycle, you should give your baby real food that you would eat. Of course, you may need to mush that up a bit if she doesn't yet have gnashers. If in doubt about weaning cycles and what to do, Susannah Olivier has a great book, *What Shall I Feed My Baby?*.

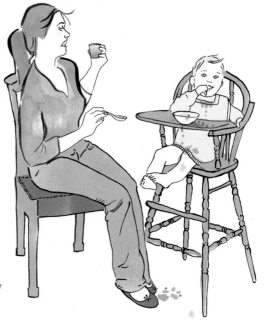

If you are back at work, then you normally have to rely on what is local to you and sometimes choices can be very hit and miss, or you have to rely on making up your own menus with a trip to the local supermarket. Of course, if you are super organised then you can bring in your own food from home. This doesn't have to mean lots of preparation. Plan to eat the same thing you had for dinner (cook extra the night before) or make a base of brown rice or wild rice or quinoa and keep adding goodies until you have a delicious salad. Include cucumber, tomatoes, lemon juice, coriander, olives, olive oil, egg, smoked fish, chicken, artichoke hearts, sun-dried tomatoes, celery – you get the idea. Obviously you don't need to put all these things together at the same time.

Help yourself

✳ Get a cleaner – even if it's only a few hours a week.

✳ Get your sister or aunt in to help you spring clean.

✳ Get a clear-it-out guru to de-clutter your space – keeping things tidy is easier when you have proper systems set up. Chris Wing of Sorted Home will help. She's an expert in general home systems, organising your wardrobe, kitchen, filing systems, but she can also research companies that can help with things like garden clearance or oven cleaning. Chris is based in London but can travel (www.sortedhome.co.uk).

This week's exercises: The 'B.I.N.G.O. and Bingo is his name-oh!' routine (this can be sung)

The exercises you are doing this week are targeting the back of your upper arms, toning into your abdominals and shaping your thighs. The benefits of doing these will not only shape and tone those troublesome areas like the bingo wings and wobbly thighs, but you will naturally raise your metabolic rate, so burning off extra calories as well as releasing the hormones that make you feel good.

I have designed this routine so you can do it with your baby in front of you, which always adds to the fun. Why not choose some nice relaxing music to perform these exercises to as they are all on the floor. For maximum benefit you need to do them slowly and in a controlled manner. So swap your fast tunes for your favourite chill-out music.

The clam

What it does: An area that many women want to tone is through their thighs and hips. So this exercise is perfect as it targets that exact area. Also, you have the bonus of engaging your abdominal muscles for support so your tummy gets a workout, too. I love this exercise as you can feel it working straightaway, so with every lift you know you are creating slim thighs. Stabilise your upper body by pulling in your tummy muscles.

What you need: A mat or towel.

1 Lie on your side on the mat with your baby near you. Keep your legs and heels together and your knees bent to a 45-degree angle.

2 Have your underneath arm extended beneath your head and the top arm relaxed out in front of you on the floor. Keep your spine in a straight line.

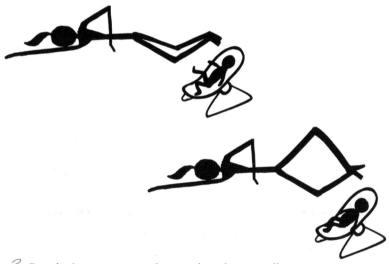

3 Breathe in to prepare and as you breathe out pull your belly button to the spine and lift the top knee, keeping your feet together and rotating at the hip. Hold for a second then slowly lower with control.

4 Do this 15 times, then rest and repeat on the same side. Turn over and work the other leg in exactly the same way.

Row the boat

What it does: This is great for working deep into your core abdominal muscle, called the transversus, which supports your back, draws in your separation and defines your waist. The exercise also tones your core muscles to give you better balance. What a fine movement it is!

What you need: A mat or towel.

1 Sit on the mat with knees bent and good upper body posture, hands resting on your knees. Have your baby on the floor in front of you.

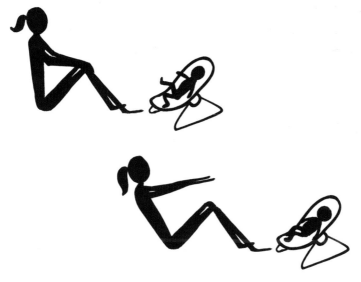

2 Take a deep breath in and as you breathe out pull in your tummy muscles and slowly lean back a couple of inches with arms extended in front of you. Hold for a couple of seconds then come back up. It is essential that as you lean back you pull your belly button to the spine and hold this until you are back to the start position. The stronger this muscle becomes, the further you will find you can lean back.

3 Repeat 10 times, rest and repeat another set.

Banish the bingo wings

What it does: This exercise is back to targeting the triceps muscle at the back of the upper arm. Yes, it's those muscles again.

What you need: A mat or towel.

1 Sit on the mat with a good posture, knees bent, feet flat on the floor and your baby close by.

2 Put your arms behind you about two hands' distance from your bottom, your elbows directly behind you and fingers pointing in towards you.

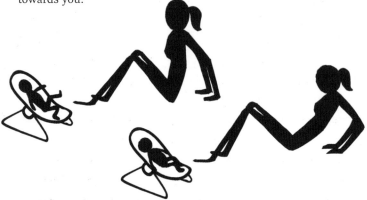

3 Take a breath in and as you breathe out pull in your tummy and slowly bend the elbows. Keeping the arms narrow as you lean back, lower your elbows several inches, hold for a couple of seconds, then slowly push back up to the start position.

4 Aim for 15, then rest and repeat another set.

Be nice to yourself

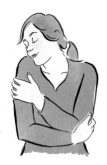

Instead of beetling about in rest hour and trying to tidy up the house, say, 'Sod it!'. No one ever died of a slightly untidy house. Put your feet up and have a rest, too – watch a trashy film or read a book. These things will make you feel human again.

Those of you at work, take your lunch break. Just

because you are a girl, don't feel guilty at taking time off to replenish. You need quality recovery time for sure.

I must say that I have recently tried to let go of having to control everything and pushing for things to happen. It is so much easier to live like this, plus you are a much nicer person to be around. The house does not have to be perfect. You are now a family and your house should look, well, a little family-fied. You know those houses where you walk in and, despite them having 25 kids and 15 dogs, the place is immaculate, with white carpets and sofas? You marvel at how they don't have melted chocolate on the cushions or dog hairs stuck to the floor. Well, all I can say is, they must be running the place like Captain Von Trapp before Maria got there. Of course, you don't want to live in a complete rubbish dump either – a happy balance and lots of yodelling is what you need. Letting go is a bit scary at first, but it is so much easier gliding through life than push, push, pushing the boulder up the hill.

You MUST eat lunch

To get the full benefit, actually stop to prepare something and don't just stuff in five stale old oatcakes and a bit of old cheese that you found lurking at the back of the fridge.

Tick list

I put my feet up (quite right too: 50 points and 3 gold stars).
I had breakfast.
I stopped for lunch – and had something filling.
I did my pram walks.
I did one of this week's exercises.

Week 7

I bet this is all second nature to you by now – I know you are just naturals at all this exercising and eating malarkey. Any problems or challenges last week? Look at the blocks – if you haven't done so already, clear out your cupboards – all those lurking packets of crisps and other num-num foods have to go (the num-nums are when you just fancy something more to eat, when secretly you know you are full). You are human for goodness sake and you will eat them, even if you don't actually like crisps. Load up with lots of healthy snacks (I like the Clearspring ones – available at any health food shop). Get loads of shopping in – I do it in bulk – with plenty of tins of chickpeas, lentils and tomatoes, and fill the freezer with frozen peas, spinach and packets of fresh fish (which you can defrost when you need it).

I hear a lot of excuses about keeping crisps and other crappy foods in for older children and that they won't eat anything else. But don't feed them rubbish (sorry to sound so militant on this point) and don't have this stuff in the house. If they have to eat it, then they can eat it with their friends (you can't generally stop them anyway). Don't make a great big fuss about not having it or it will become a great big family thing – in your house, it just isn't there.

This week's exercises: The weight-less weights routine

For this week all the exercises are performed standing up. You will be toning your abdominals, shoulders, triceps, waist and inner and outer thighs as well as lifting your buttocks.

To make this week fun, you can train with your baby so I suggest that you put some bright long ribbons around your hand weights. Your baby can focus on the colours and as long as she is positioned near you as you exercise, she can be tickled as you move up and down with the weights. You can then burn off even more calories by running around the room with your toddler after she's tried to prise the ribbons off your weights.

Ballet butt with weights

What it does: This one works on your buttocks, hips, tummy *and* inner and outer thighs. Do not let your knees shoot over the line of your toes.

What you need: A hand weight or small full bottles of water (plus your baby).

1 Holding the weight in front of you in both hands, palms facing in towards your body, stand with your feet wider than a hip-width distance and have your toes at a 45-degree angle. Keep your upper body straight and knees soft.

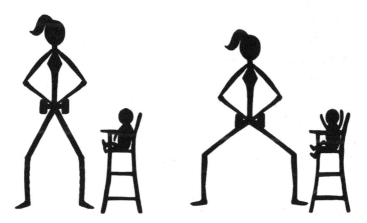

2 Take a deep breath in and as you breathe out pull in your tummy muscles and lower yourself by bending through the knees, keeping your upper body straight. Lower your hips several inches, hold and then slowly push back up.

3 Aim for 20 reps, rest and repeat another set.

Twist and shout

What it does: Quite simply, this one tones your waist muscles.

What you need: A hand weight or small full bottles of water.

1 Holding the weight with both hands, stand tall with good posture. Raise your arms in front of you, palms facing down, knees soft and tummy pulled in.

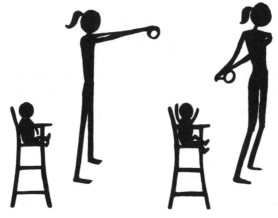

2 Without moving your knees or hips, slowly rotate your upper body leading though the arms to one side. Hold for a second, then rotate to the other side. Keep your abs pulled in and be sure to feel this working in your waist. If you can't, you may need to reach around a little further. Keep everything slow and controlled.

3 Do 20 times, rest and repeat another set.

Water-skiing fantasy

What it does: This is a fantastic exercise to give you sleek and sexy shoulders and, at the same time, you can get toning those tummy muscles by keeping them pulled in.

What you need: Hand weights or small full bottles of water.

1 Holding the weights together in front of you at hip height, stand with good posture, feet a hip-width distance apart, knees soft and your palms facing the ground.

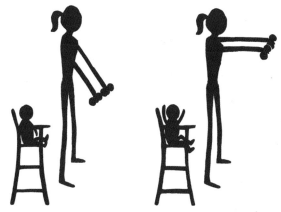

2 Breathing in, pull in your tummy and lift your arms to shoulder height. Hold for a second then slowly lower, breathing out at the same time. Keep your tummy pulled in to support your back and keep all movement slow and controlled.

3 Aim to do 20 times, rest and repeat another set.

Be nice to yourself

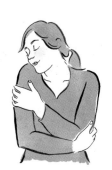

When you are out on your pram walk and if you live in a town, go and treat yourself to a delicious juice. If you can make your own at home, then combine orange, mint, lime and pomegranate ... mmmm, lovely. Try out various combos from *Power Juices – Super Drinks* by Steve Meyerowitz (Kensington Publishing Corp).

You MUST clean out the cupboards of all lurking num-nums
Go on – you'll be pleased when you have done it.

Tick list

I have varied my breakfast all week (10 extra points).

I did my pram walk.

I looked in the mirror and just saw my good points (50 extra points).

I put my feet up and read a trashy magazine (and didn't feel guilty).

I kissed my partner and told him I loved him.

Week 8

Can you believe it? At the end of this week you will have been doing something about your health and your exercise for *two whole months*. You must be feeling a whole lot better by now.

This week's exercises: The golden medal routine

The exercises you will be doing this week will be toning through your shoulders, abdominals and buttocks. As these are all big muscle groups you have the added bonus of burning off even more calories.

Crouching breathing tiger

What it does: This one works deep into your core muscles. It's a simple exercise where you just pull in your tummy.

What you need: A mat or towel.

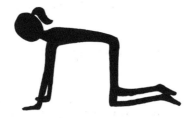

1 Kneel on the mat on all-fours. Keeping your back in a straight line and your elbows slightly bent to avoid locking them out. Look at the floor.

2 Take a deep breath in and as you breathe out draw your navel up towards your spine without moving or arching your back. Hold for 6 seconds, then slowly release. Repeat.

3 Aim for 10, then rest and repeat the set.

Continental loo

What it does: Tones your buttocks for a perky bottom as well as your thighs and abs. Plus, this is a great way of increasing your metabolic rate.

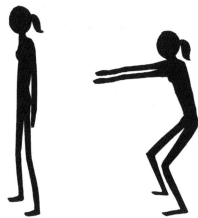

1 Stand with good posture and your feet a shoulder width apart and knees soft. Bend your legs and lower your body as if you are going to sit on a chair. At the same time, raise your arms in front of you, parallel to the floor.

2 Be sure not to let your knees go over the line of your toes, return to standing, driving the weight through your heels, thighs and then bottom.

3 Aim for 20, then rest and repeat another set.

Lying chest flyer

What it does: Helps to tone up your bust line and gives you a curvier and sexier shape.

What you need: A mat or towel and hand weights or small full bottles of water.

1 Lie on your back on the mat with your knees bent and feet flat on the floor. Holding your weights in both hands, palms facing up, rest your arms out to the side of your body on the floor. They should be in line or slightly lower than your bust.

2 Take a deep breath in, pull in your tummy and lift your arms from either side. Keep the elbows slightly bent with palms facing each other until they meet. Hold for a second then slowly lower to start position.

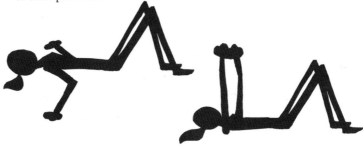

3 Aim to do this 20 times, then rest for a minute and perform a second set.

Be nice to yourself

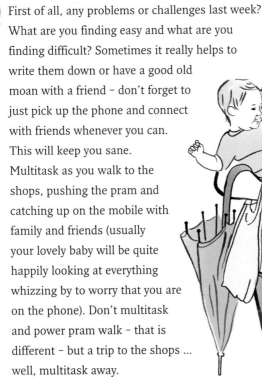

First of all, any problems or challenges last week? What are you finding easy and what are you finding difficult? Sometimes it really helps to write them down or have a good old moan with a friend – don't forget to just pick up the phone and connect with friends whenever you can. This will keep you sane. Multitask as you walk to the shops, pushing the pram and catching up on the mobile with family and friends (usually your lovely baby will be quite happily looking at everything whizzing by to worry that you are on the phone). Don't multitask and power pram walk – that is different – but a trip to the shops ... well, multitask away.

You MUST get a new habit

Habits do take a long time to establish but once you have a new, positive habit it tends to stick. We usually think of habits as negative things – like a smoking habit or drug habit – but they can be positive, too ... like shopping (oops!), I mean like having breakfast everyday. By now this should be well tucked in under your belt of things to do in the morning. You see? You don't even remember the days when you used to skip it. And if you are not doing breakfast then I haven't been nagging you enough.

Give it a rest

Remember, don't get too carried away. Don't do too much toning – take a break.

Exercise is also about making it a habit – that means something that glides into your day without you making a supreme effort. You do feel so much better moving than not moving. Humans were not designed to sit looking at computer screens all day or to be slobbing in front of the TV. We are designed as moving machines and if you don't oil the bits by moving them, they will stiffen up and stop working.

I know you are busy but add in one new positive habit this week. It could be:

✳ Putting on your make-up to face the world instead of just steaming out of the house without a thought.

✳ Just drinking alcohol once a week (for you brave souls who drink more than this!).

✳ Writing thank you letters as soon as you need to rather than waiting six weeks.

✳ Stopping for tea and putting your feet up.

Tick list

I got a new habit.
I ate breakfast.
I did the pram walking.
I did all the exercises for this week.
I smiled.
I left the cleaning, so the house is not perfectly tidy.

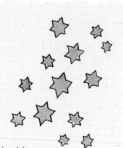

To infinity and beyond

How do you keep this all going in a forever-type way? By now you should have started laying down great foundations for life and instead of it all being an effort and something you are having to try very hard to keep up by massively concentrating on it all this great nutrition and exercise should be a way of life. I have said it before and I will say it again, you don't have to be perfect so don't stress about the details. Some days are going to go according to plan and some days are not. Sometimes, for whatever reason, you might get into a loop of drinking too much, eating too much or not doing enough exercise. We all go through these phases – accept them. Rope yourself in and try to form new habits that stick.

I confess that I am not manic about formal exercise (going to the gym for me would be a complete nightmare – all those other girls in tight lycra showing off their perfect bodies). So, if this is you and you hate exercise, just up your activity levels and concentrate on getting your stomach area back in trim ... and keep on moving. Let's face it, there's no chance of sitting on your butt when you're chasing a little bean around the place, is there?

If you are keen on exercise, Lucy's programme is fantastic and do-able. The trick is to build exercise into your everyday existence. I get up in my exercise gear, take my daughter to nursery and then pride stops me from collecting her in my exercise gear. Between dropping her and collection I will have to have done at least something. You feel so much better emotionally, physically, mentally and spiritually for exercising.

Keeping in the groove

If you need help, think on these pointers:

Food

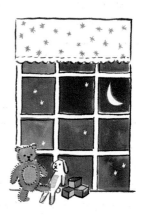

* If everything turns to filth and the whole of your good habit basis collapses, go back and get the breakfast 'right'.
* Get inspiration by looking at some books on nutrition – just look at the pictures, don't get into the fine print (unless you enjoy that, of course).
* Revise the Rules and see what you are actually working to.
* Never weigh yourself!
* Boring, boring, boring, but watch that you are not eating a *huge* portion at each meal.

Life

* Don't get overwhelmed – concentrate on the *now* today and the things that you can change.
* You don't have to have a perfectly tidy house.
* Plan for tomorrow, but don't *worry* about tomorrow.
* Get help. Ask for it – generally people are not telepathic.
* Choose to be happy and fulfilled – don't expect a lightning bolt to arrive from heaven and bestow joy upon you.

The universe

* Be grateful for what you have got rather than looking around at what you haven't got. You may be surprised to learn that actually you are doing OK!

Keep it up . . . exercise-wise

The following programmes can be followed on an on-going basis as you can repeat them for up to three weeks at a time before moving on, then start over again. As you get fitter, you could combine two programmes together.

For toning, work on the exercises used previously, but try to do four exercises at a time instead of the three as you progress in fitness.

First infinity routine

Power walk four times a week, each for 20 minutes

Curtsey to the queen (see page 129)

Wonder woman waist (see page 133)

Continental loo (see page 155)

I must, I must (see page 89)

Second infinity routine

Power walk, swim or cycle: three sessions a week – one for 30 minutes and the other two for 25 minutes

The clam (see page 146)

Twist and shout (see page 152)

Ballet butt (see page 134)

Wonder woman waist (see page 133)

Third infinity routine

Power walk, swim or cycle: aim this week to do four sessions but only for 20 minutes each

Lying chest flyer (see pages 155–6)

Row the boat (see page 147)

Kiss your baby and leg lift (see page 141)

Heel taps (see page 91)

Fourth infinity routine

Power walk, swim or cycle: aim for three sessions all for 30 minutes

Yes, miss! Yes, miss! (see pages 134–5)

Row the boat (see page 147)

Wonder woman waist (see page 133)

Continental loo (see page 155)

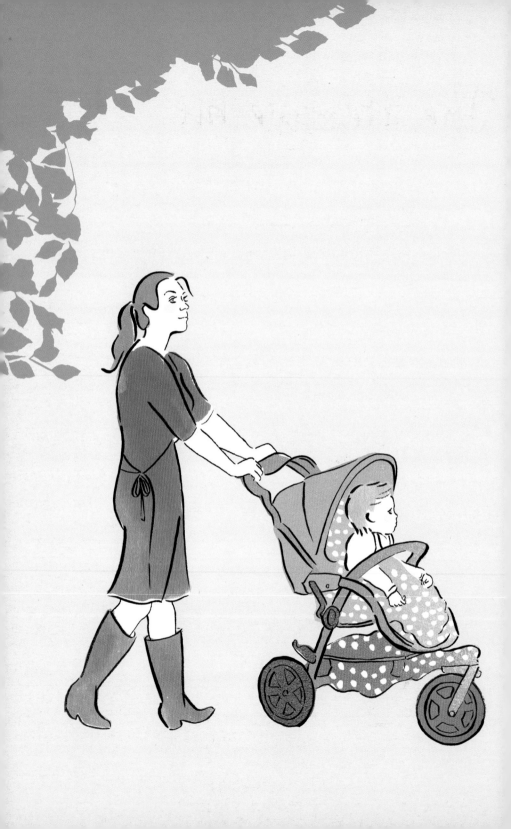

The lifestyle bit

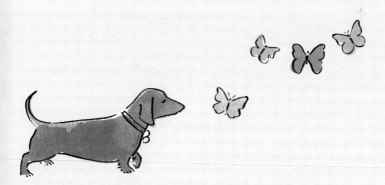

And now we are two

I have a very nice friend who has just given birth to number two. She is such a sweet person but keeps on insisting that she has recently turned into the devil incarnate. Among some of the issues that are transforming her character, she claims that:

* She has been really, really crabby with her partner.
* She has no patience with number one son.
* She is completely knackered and on the verge of feeling depressed.
* She feels like giving up and running away.
* She feels like giving one of the children up to social services (not really, but nearly).

If you, too, feel like this, then think on.

Be nice to yourself

* You deserve to feel knackered. You are up feeding in the night and with a new foreign object that you might not have bonded with yet. It takes time to get to know each other. So don't feel guilty if you are not a 'gushy mummy'.
* The baby has stolen your vitamins and minerals. Make sure you are taking a good multi-vitamin and possibly some extra zinc (which could help to ward off depression). See pages 64-9.
* Get some help. Can your mum or a friend step in so that you can get some rest?
* Do you have a good nursery you can book child number one into to free yourself up sometimes during the week?
* Go out! Not straightaway, maybe, but finding some adult time for you and your partner is vital.

Time

The one luxury that evaporates practically overnight is time. I say overnight but once you are past the very early days and you are not like a constant milk-machine and are not so wiped out, you might have a bit more time than you thought. Especially if you were used to working in an office before getting pregnant. When the baby is kipping, you might actually put up your feet and read a magazine, quietly read a book or take a long relaxing bath (rather than manically cleaning the kitchen).

Of course, the toddler stage is a whole new ball game ... 'ball' and 'game' being favourite activities. Others include tipping make-up bag down the loo, posting only set of keys down street drain or picking up the only item in the room that could potentially electrocute the little love. Stuffing Panda Bear into the dishwasher comes a close second.

What you might not have any more is acres of luscious, luxurious, lovely time that stretches ahead, like a cool balmy summer's day. But what you do have is small snatches of time. Little pockets. And this is a load better than nothing. Seizing the moment is key, because you often can't plan these little oases of space – they just appear. Of course they are better planned, these snippets of glorious peace, but snatching them comes a close second. The temptation is to do everything properly. Proper time to go to the gym, proper time to do some yoga. A round trip to the gym might be a few hours, and while the crèche is a fabulous idea, what if you get all the way there and it is full? And when are you really going to get a few hours? Once a week?

When your mum pops round, use her (nicely girls!). She wants to help you and she really wants to have a moment to herself with her grandchild. She is dying for you not to be so hands-on so she can show you how it all should be done. So grab your trainers and head outside. Take this book with you and actually do some of the exercises that Lucy has laid out for you. Don't try to do *all* of them. Some is just great. Plan what you could do every day in just 15–20 minutes of time and when this elusive door opens, you will be ready and raring to go.

Useful things to do with 15 minutes

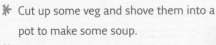

* Have a kip – go with it. You might need to take a rest. Do *not* feel guilty.
* Go for a gentle jog round the block.
* Cut up some veg and shove them into a pot to make some soup.
* Give yourself a facial.
* Have a long shower and shave your legs.
* Do some of Lucy's exercises.
* Put some make-up on. It will make you look better even if you feel knackered.
* Order your shopping online rather than struggling to the supermarket.

Be nice to yourself

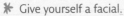

* Time slots will appear and disappear just as fast – so make use of them. Seize the moment.
* You don't have to do everything properly to get great results. Do what you can.

Boredom

You might think that the last thing that would scupper your new body programme would be boredom. Boredom, I hear you cry. Are you mad? Have you seen the amount of *stuff* I have to get through in a day? Bored? I don't get time to be bored. Well, before you go off on one, let me explain.

Some of you will have looked forward to the new regime that this bundle of life has bestowed on you – an event that you have looked forward to, in fact, since you were a tiny girl. Playing with your dolls back then, you told yourself that one day you would have your own family of a girl and a boy. This glowing vision is, of course, all wrapped up in fluffy bows with tiny rabbits and other furry woodland animals looking on and talking amongst themselves, exchanging loving but knowing looks. And now, years later the dream has come true and, like all dreams, there are really good bits and, well, not so good bits. How you see what is good and what is bad depends on you. Some people are able to cope with the good, the bad and the ugly. They glide through it, but for some people the reality of the sleepless nights and the soggy nappies is not the dream that they signed up for. The struggle is that you love your tiny love-packet but you are not so keen on the full-time admin. You can get to resent the disturbed nights, the endless washing, the grime and the toys.

For those of you that have been working full-time in a career, being a full-time domestic might seem great at first. Anything to get away from the dreaded emails and the boss, but in the end you start to miss, even crave, adult conversation that doesn't involve someone else's kid being the next Einstein.

And when you were in your previous life you would scoff at those folk who turned on daytime telly. The morning news is different, you tell yourself, and before you know it you have watched the Oprah equivalent that follows. Boy, do some people have complicated lives. Whoops! You can't believe you spent the whole of the baby's morning nap learning about a one-legged lesbian who has been reunited with her long-lost family. As you wipe away the tears you realise you are addicted.

You accept the deal that your job while you are off work is to look after your baby while your partner brings in the bacon. However, if this was your real job, you'd be in the boss's office for a little chat (next time written warning) because you forgot to make any dinner again – well, you didn't actually forget, you ran out of time. You can see from the look on your beloved's face that he can't believe that you ran out of time ... the 'What does she *do* all day?' face gives the game away

The boredom and the biscuit tin are inextricably linked – the two Bs. You are not really hungry you are just bored.

Be nice to yourself

✳ Don't keep biscuits in the house or other false friends.

✳ Hook up with other mums. Find a new best-mate mum who you can be really honest with and not pretend that all is rosy in the garden if it really isn't.

✳ Tell your partner to bog off if he gives you one of those 'What *has* she been doing all day?' looks. Let him do it for a while (mind you, the house would look like it had been burgled by the end of a day with him in charge). Men can't multitask, as we all know. Find me one that can look after a baby, cook the meals *and* have a tidy house.

Change in status

The biggest thing to hit my friend Jill between the eyeballs about motherhood is how, before she was a mother, she was *something*. Now don't get me wrong, being a mother is great, wonderful, rewarding, challenging, but before being a mum she had a career. A role where she was in control and now she has a job where a tiny fluff ball is running the show. Before, she had respect and power. People listened (or at least were polite enough to pretend they were listening). Now people sometimes actually don't pay any attention to her at all – even when she has got something quite important to say.

Camilla is the president of her resident's association and wanted to arrange some finance with her bank manager to do some major structural work on the building (she took a break from a major city company of accountants to have her baby). She went along with her Polish builder (as he happened to offer her a lift). The bank manager totally ignored everything she was saying (even the spreadsheets she had brought) and

Be nice to yourself

* Try to retain something of the old you even if it means getting a baby-sitter in once a week for half a day.
* Don't dress like a hippo when you go out and for goodness sake put your slap on. There's no excuse for becoming down at heel (despite all the excuses).
* Tell the bank manager or any other similar characters where to stuff it.

conducted the whole conversation at the bloke, which was totally lost on him anyway, as he doesn't speak English. In fact, Camilla is convinced that she has an invisible cloak on and when she speaks it all gets translated into 'Bimbo'.

Isolation

Wow! The baby is finally here and settled in and the stork has flapped off. The flowers and the balloons have wilted. The cards have stopped arriving. The visitors have trailed off. Your chap is back to work.

Right, better start making some good plans about how the day is going to go, you say to yourself, but by lunchtime the whole plan has dissolved in tears. You didn't realise that it took so long to breastfeed. The baby fell asleep halfway through. You fell asleep when the baby was sleeping – think how much you could have done? The house is a complete tip. As you have never actually waited for the washing machine to finish its cycle you didn't know that it takes about two hours. OK, it wasn't your fault that you only managed one load. Have you seen how much kit these babies get through? You have even started to take on super-slob mother tactics and turn the babysuits inside out to make them last an extra day. As for your clothes, old slug tracks (where junior has wiped her nose down the back of your T-shirt), are the least of your worries. Tomato pasta down your trousers. You really hope no one will notice. You are contributing to global warming single handedly with all the washing cycles you are doing and as for the nappies you are getting through. You have actually started to panic about landfill. Very seriously.

You plan to go to the shops. It takes four hours to get out of the house because you keep forgetting things. And your flat is on the top floor. The bag, the nappies, the bottles (easier if you only have to take your own boobs with you – saves all sorts of issues), the emergency oatcakes, the wipes, the toys, the extra clothes just in case, oh and the pushchair. OK, finally at the car and then you have to work out how that blasted car seat buckle works – it only slots together if you know the secret. Combo. Fiddle. Fiddle. Fiddle. Fiddle. Baby gets cheesed off and starts yelling. Getting stressed now, it actually takes you a record 15 minutes to get the baby strapped in. Your back is killing you with all that unnatural bending over. Down to the supermarket to do the family shop – now, how is this going to work? Shopping, baby, paying and then getting back in the car, where the baby has a meltdown moment. ARRGGGH!

It is quite normal to feel very isolated. If you have previously been working, all this domestic bliss is quite a shock. You do feel like you are losing control, especially if you are used to being in control.

Be nice to yourself

* Don't do this by yourself. Plan an expedition out every day that doesn't involve the car.
* Invite *anyone* over for tea on a regular basis.
* Go and have tea in your fave café.
* Accept that you will feel lonely and miss adult conversation, but that phases pass and you will get your life back.

Growing-up

Another hard thing about parenthood, if you let it be hard, of course, is the mourning of the old self. All the things you left behind. The lounging in bed on a Sunday with the papers, the meals out, the friends over until four in the morning, the spontaneous trips to Barcelona ... OK, how many of those things did you really do anyway? I think our generation find it hard to move onto the other stages of life without holding on. We don't have to be the dowdy mum-type in a tweed skirt, twin set, pearls and a perm. My granny looked like a granny aged 40. A lot of us are thinking about having our first baby at 40 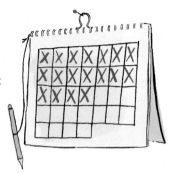 these days – how things have changed. A body piercing? A boob job? Anything to deny the passing of our youth and stages of our life.

You have to experience loss before you can experience gain. So in letting go of your past life, you gain a whole lot of other great stuff, but it's hard to let go of most of the old stuff first. Don't be like the monkey with his hand in the jar of nuts – in grabbing the nuts he is stuck, but in letting go, he is free.

Be nice to yourself

✳ Try and accept where you are now and you'll be much happier.

Putting others first

Women are really good at playing lots of different roles in life and now you have another one to add to your repertoire – motherhood. Boy, do you have a lot of hats on now. It would be really fun if you really did have to wear different hats for different roles, but sadly this type of fun is just make-believe and the dressing-up box. Wouldn't it be great if, like a cartoon character, each hat meant that you could live a different, more exciting life and it transported you to a different land and experience? Just like Mr Benn. Back to earth and more realistically, you wear the hat of being a partner, a lover, an aunt, a sister, a homemaker, an employee, a business owner – and now the biggest one of them all – Mum, Mummy, Mamma, Mom – or as I am, Ammah.

Suddenly, the overwhelming responsibility of motherhood can strike us between the eyes Here is a tiny, wee, defenceless little fluffy chick of a thing – and he is totally dependent on us for grub, comfort, warmth, and love – the only things he does pretty effectively by himself are pooing and sleeping. Good skills for life, I think you'll agree.

The temptation is to lose yourself in the trying to be Mrs Wonderful for everyone else. What are their needs? How can I make them more comfortable? What can I do to help? In being needed, it can bolster our own sense of self-worth and sense of who we think we should be. 'If they need me, I must be really important.' This is an illusion as eventually you just get cheesed off that you are running around after everyone, picking up socks and Mr Panda, who has got wedged down the side of the washing machine, without so much as a please or a thank you. In my experience, men really do not appreciate a tidy house anyway, so you are wasting your time.

You are too busy now to play all these roles as perfectly as before. Remember that most relationships should be give *and* take, but do you ever get the impression that some relationships are all about the take? It does always seem to be you that makes the phone call to your brother, your uncle and their aunt, and it's you that pops round as a shoulder to cry on for your mates. Well, things have got to change. You might lose a few casualties on the way – maybe you don't get to speak to your brother as often as you would like – but it is a two-way street and all these people you have helped have to help you now. It's time to pull in the favours. Ask for help. You can't do it all by yourself, Mrs Martyr. Us women have a tendency to think that the more we look like a wistful Joan of Arc, mopping our brows and looking up to the heavens for inspiration, the more someone is going to notice how absolutely wonderful we are and how hard we work. The bad news is that no one is paying the least bit attention to this tactic and it is largely falling on deaf ears and blind mice. Forget it. You need to be very clear in how you ask for help. Hinting will not cut the mustard.

Be nice to yourself

* Ask for help – telepathy is tricky to master.
* Pull in the favours – it's pay-back time!
* Dropping heavy hints about how hard you work doesn't work.
* Don't play the martyr – it's not a good look. Who was Joan of Arc's stylist anyway? (That hair ... really.)

Tiredness — the death of all good intentions

Now you have decided to get a grip and do something about you, for you – well done! The great thing about looking after your health and fitness is that it will make you feel great about yourself and look fantastic. You will have never-ending energy, vitality and a whoosh of life-giving power. Well I would say that, wouldn't I?

Can you imagine that? The answer is that I guess it depends when you are reading these words. No one prepares you for the overwhelming tiredness of being a mother – in fact, in the old days no one told the unattached (unmarried!) lady anything about childbirth or motherhood for fear of putting us girls off the whole thing – an unspoken code. Of course, that code has been blasted out of the water nowadays and we are treated to blow-by-blow descriptions of every last feature in every medium. I am sure that there must be blogs out there dedicated to this very topic.

After the exhaustion, exhilaration and deflation of giving birth, unless you are lucky enough to have a hands-on mother, friend or can pay for a maternity nurse, then all too quickly you are expected just to get on with it. That means looking after junior with no instruction manual. Cooking, doing the shopping and getting dressed (you that is, not the baby) can all seem overwhelming and unless you had the forethought to get organised before, then your systems, as they are, will bulge underneath the new pressures and definitely start creaking at the seams.

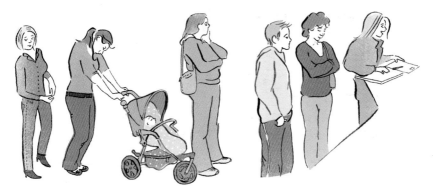

This is what I call treacle tiredness, when you have to drag yourself about like your legs are trapped in something very sticky and gooey – like a fly stuck on a piece of flypaper. The more you struggle, the more tired you feel – heavy feet, itchy eyes, mouth like the bottom of a parrots cage – so unfair when you haven't even touched a drop.

You will get used to your new lifestyle

Don't despair. First of all, it does usually get better. You get more used to your new life as you understand that your baby will normally get through the night without you rushing up to his room every three minutes to hold a mirror under his nostrils to check if he is still breathing. You do eventually stop with the obsessional checking of the lights on the baby unit, and one day you will stop holding the monitor so close to your face that it practically burns your ears to check if he is breathing. Is that breathing or not? Not sure, better rush up with the mirror and check.

You will get your sleep back

Once the night feeds have stopped, this will happen – unless, of course you are unlucky. We only had to think about my nephew and he would by some telepathic power be up and yelling on full lung capacity until he was really quite old. But he is 12 now and sleeping like a baby. So take heart!

You will recover your energy

The day will come when you feel the bounce come back – especially if you look after your diet and exercise – however gently you ease yourself into a regime. I have friends who lived on takeaways for the first few months and they felt and looked awful. Of course the more awful they felt the more they craved crap food. On crappy junk food, your

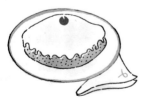

blood sugar will crash, leaving you craving more. You then get in a cycle of tiredness that you can't get out of.

A wonderfully supportive partner is key. Even really simple meals that he can whack in the oven as soon as he is home are going to make a huge difference to your energy levels – food like grilled fish, roast chicken, even beans on toast (organic, of course!).

Just know that this tiredness will pass and it will all get better and if it's been your excuse not to get started on getting into shape, then so be it. Don't bash yourself up. Take it one day at a time. Start to plan to get your energy back by dealing with the small things first, rather than the big.

Be nice to yourself

* Go to bed earlier – get your partner onside on this one.
* If you really are drop-dead knockout tired, it's worth a visit to the doctor to check if you are iron deficient or get them to check your thyroid is on full power.
* Drink plenty of water, even though it can be difficult to remember drinking with the new regime – dehydration makes you tired.
* Coffee makes you even more tired and if you are breastfeeding might make your baby wired.
* Alcohol – you might crave it (another blood sugar drop) but, boy, is it bad news either the next day or when you can't sleep. If you are breastfeeding, it can't be a healthy product for your baby's tiny liver either.
* Know that this tiredness will pass, but start making adjustments to your routine now – small changes to get your energy back. Begin with fresh food and fresh air.

Eating out

That first euphoria of motherhood – all those invitations out. Friends.
The pop of the champagne cork and it was so easy, just popping little
Mary into the Moses basket and setting off. And wasn't she good?
She just slept and looked really sweet. Going out in those days
was a doddle! Just discreetly getting out a boob or sticking her on
the bottle was a joy. That's if you had the energy and had something
to wear. Feeling that the only thing that fitted was the vast pair of
elephant-like tracksuit bottoms with attractive drawstring 'active'
waistband device is never great for the self-esteem. Even the elephant
didn't want to wear them. Eating
out. Remember that?

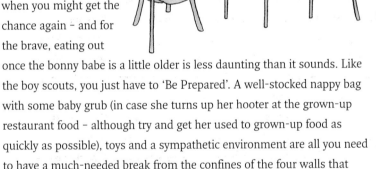

   Well, make the
effort. In the early
days, do try to get out
there as much as
possible, you don't know
when you might get the
chance again – and for
the brave, eating out
once the bonny babe is a little older is less daunting than it sounds. Like
the boy scouts, you just have to 'Be Prepared'. A well-stocked nappy bag
with some baby grub (in case she turns up her hooter at the grown-up
restaurant food – although try and get her used to grown-up food as
quickly as possible), toys and a sympathetic environment are all you need
to have a much-needed break from the confines of the four walls that
have become your home.

   More to the point, don't let eating out be an excuse for what I call
'The Magic Harry Potter Cloak' of invisible behaviour. Once you are out,
the temptation is to go totally nuts – this is a 'treat' after all. You might
not be eating for two any more, but who cares? Just this one time will not
make a difference, surely? You are freeeee ... that scrumptious bread
basket with the olive oil, that one glass of bubbly that turns into four, the
pudding that you never have ... hmmmm, quite a blow out. Good news!

The Magic Harry Potter cloak protects you from any weight gain or hangover. Until you realise there never was any magic cloak, and boy do you feel rough at 4am when the siren wails from junior strike up.

Rules are there to be broken . . .

... but don't break all of them at once. Choose the rule you want to break. Just one. Easy little compromises are to give the breadbasket a skip. Just look the waiter in the eye and say that you would like the delicious olive and pine nut ciabatta bread that was imported fresh from the Tuscan countryside out of your life, thank you. Look, it's not your fault. When your blood sugar is low, adapting to going through treacle tiredness, the bread is crying out to be eaten. Mad though it sounds, have a snack of an oatcake with some cottage cheese or hummus before you go, then you are not in the situation where you would just eat anything when you get there.

Passing on the potatoes is also possible – order fresh green veg on the side to fill you up. Just say 'no' to sauce – the plainer the food, the better. Gravy is a hard one to resist – so don't – just make sure you have less of it. A glass of wine? Have you tried a spritzer? I know it's blindingly obvious, but clear soups, salads, fish and chicken are generally less dangerous choices. And pudding – by all means order a dessert, but ask the waiter to bring enough spoons for you all to share. Try not to look wistful as your crème brulée disappears to the far end of the table. It wasn't yours, remember, you were sharing.

As long as the restaurant is happy to have a baby in their midst, don't compromise in choosing a place the baby might like. Within reason, go for somewhere you want to eat and a place where it is more or less possible to stick to your resolutions.

Be nice to yourself

* Go out – even for a short time without the baby (obviously get a baby-sitter).
* Use some lavender bath oil, which is great for relaxation.
* Flowers will cheer you up – drop a hint to your partner.

Going on holiday

First of all, good luck! Now you know why the Beckhams have their own private jet. You never knew you needed so much stuff; travel cot, enough nappies to sink a battleship, monitor (or the PPU – paranoid parent unit) and that is before you have packed 200 changes of clothes. And you never know, it might snow in Majorca in May, so better bring the baby Artic gear in case.

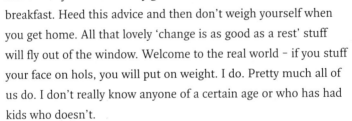

Again, the Harry Potter Cloak rule applies on hols – you can do a lot of damage in two weeks. Often when your routine is broken, it really is very difficult to stick to a regime. Do your best, though. Be nice to yourself, but don't use the holiday as an excuse to go bonkers. If all else fails, just make sure you have a really good breakfast. Heed this advice and then don't weigh yourself when you get home. All that lovely 'change is as good as a rest' stuff will fly out of the window. Welcome to the real world – if you stuff your face on hols, you will put on weight. I do. Pretty much all of us do. I don't really know anyone of a certain age or who has had kids who doesn't.

So, if you have stuffed your face don't worry about it once you are back; just get back into your normal routine and everything will be fine in a couple of weeks. Stop any negative chat. You had a nice time, but now you are home it's time to get back on the horse. Besides, the holiday snaps have been downloaded and that is the last time you are going to be wearing that huge Demis Roussos kaftan to hide your stomach.

The only concession to faddiness I make when planning a holiday is taking my own breakfast with me. I take my wheat-free muesli and some rice milk in the suitcase. This is particularly useful at least for the first few days while you get the lay of the land because then breakfast is sorted. Getting your blood sugar right from the start of the day is really important. Once breakfast is taken care of, you are much more likely to make better choices for the rest of the day.

Holidays are also one of the only times where 'full-time' help with a partner is usually more forthcoming, because he is there and not at work. Have a discussion before you go about each having some time to pursue individual goals – he might want to do kite surfing and you might need some time off from the baby to do your daily walking and exercise while listening to your iPod. Men are usually a lot better at expressing what they need to do, while women sometimes try to fit in to be nice ... not surprisingly, this can lead to a lot of general chuntering of unexpressed frustration: 'Why am I left with the baby again, while he's off having fun?' Well, to be fair to your beloved, he hasn't probably developed the telepathic gene yet, so tell him what you need and want out of the holiday before you go. Make sure you have similar holiday aims or you could find that you are looking for different ideas of time away from home. If you are not going on hols with your partner, taking a willing girlfriend might be the solution – being on duty by yourself 24/7 is no picnic.

Holidaying with your wee one, I should flag up at this point, is no way compatible with any of the following words: relaxed, chilled-out, break, reading a book/newspaper. Have fun anyway!

Be nice to yourself

* Pack your own breakfast.
* Remember that the Magic Harry Potter Cloak doesn't exist.
* Don't beat yourself up if you go nuts – just get back on the horse once you are home.
* Delegate some childcare to your partner and run for the hills!

And now we are three

I am sure you are used to your lovely smiling, supportive partner helping you with everything in your life – understanding, caring, protective and loyal is how you used to describe him. What you certainly didn't sign up for was the Incredible Hulk or the incredible sulk more like. Blimey O'Reilly, what has got into him lately?

Are you used to having those little loving, intimate moments when he comes in through the door from work? You throw your arms around his neck as he swings you round in an affectionate embrace (well, maybe not). But nowadays he comes home just as the baby is in the bath and of course you can't just leave junior there up to his armpit in suds (obviously that's the first thing they teach you, isn't it?). Actually, to be truthful, you didn't even hear the door go you were so into gurgling sweet nothings into the baby's beautiful ears, blowing raspberries and squeezing out the water from Olly the octopus's bottom that you didn't even register that it must be coming home time. The next thing you know, your partner has dumped his coat and is going out for a run. Not even a word. 'Something I said?', you wonder?

I know they (other mums) tell you this the whole time, but men really do seem to have their noses put out of joint when junior comes along. I am sure there are all sorts of complicated reasons as to why Mr Grumpy comes out to play. No longer top lion, perhaps – a new cub to lead the pack eventually? Is it the way you look dreamily in to your baby's eyes, sighing – you haven't looked into anyone else's eyes with that loving dopey look since you met your partner, getting it together after too many tequila sunrises. Could the old emerald-eyed demon have popped into his head? Mr J for Jealousy? Surely not! Surely your partner understands that baby-love is not the same thing at all.

Also, life changes forever when you have a baby and with the change comes the realisation of responsibility – how much did they say the school fees for Eton were? Nothing but the *best* for my boy. Actually, let's start at the beginning. How much is the Montessori Nursery a month. What? That much? Better make some more cash and be a little more serious about the job. Before Baby, your partner thought that if he didn't like the boss or the coffee he could just walk out any time he liked, but now, well, he has responsibilities now, doesn't he?

And actually you haven't exactly been sweetness and light now we are on the subject. You have been just a little crabbier and a bit snappier than usual what with the disturbed nights and not knowing if that little cough your baby has developed is TB or not. So give your partner a break. He is trying to adapt to a whole new way of being, too, and it can be stressful for everyone. The most important thing is not to take it personally. It is the stress talking. Phases pass in your baby's life and it all does become much easier. I promise. And besides, you need your partner on board to help you reclaim your body, mind and sanity. So a little understanding all round is called for.

Be nice to yourself

✱ Remember that a new baby is stressful for everyone – including the baby.

✱ Random shouting and unreasonable behaviour will pass.

✱ Be careful to make a great big fuss of your lovely man – make him feel that he hasn't been shoved to the bottom of the pile (even if he has).

Lazy Dad/Helpful Dad

Men are always saying that they can't win. Well, they are right – for once. You can be helped to reach your health goals either by the most helpful man in the world or the laziest. Now how does that work?

We all dream of having the perfect partner. The one who has cooked dinner, fed the baby, drawn your deliciously hot bath filled with rose petals, essential oils and asses milk. This, of course, is brilliant because while your delightfully helpful chap is attending to all the chores, you can have your trainers on and be half way to completing a ten-mile run or doing 20 press-ups, all at the same 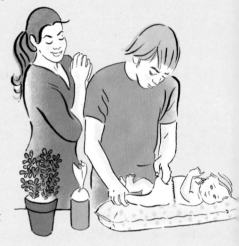 time. Well on your way to completing your health goals certainly. If you do have this incredible man in your life, for goodness sake don't let him out of your sight.

A helpful partner is great, but you must take the opportunity and take the time he is giving you without feeling guilty and certainly don't apply the freed-up time elsewhere. Guilt is one of woman's most destructive scupperers. He loves you, he is giving you permission to do your stuff, he is happy if you are happy, so get out there and do something. Don't make excuses and remember that 15 minutes to do something towards your health and wellbeing is great. Just doing some of the exercises, some of the nutrition and some of the other ideas is much better than doing nothing at all. You don't need an hour's luxury of time to make a huge difference, you just need consistency and stickability doing small things, but over and over again to build habit. If you are worried about a payback, I am sure you will think of something, but don't promise anything that you haven't got the energy for right now!

If you are turning green at this point and wondering how you ended up with Mr Slobby Unhelpful don't be too hard on your smug sister's Mr Perfect. You could actually profit hugely from this state of affairs. Yes, you will have to run around like a headless chicken trying to fit everything in. Running up and down the stairs, doing all the shopping, cleaning and looking after the baby full time is a wonderful way to work off all those extra calories and trim your legs at the same time. So next time you are cursing your bad luck for picking the laziest man in the Universe, just think how lucky you are!

* If your partner is helpful, thoughtful, loving and gives you time for yourself – don't let him out of the house.
* But lazy man is a blessing in disguise for there's no time to sit on your bum and doing everything will work off extra calories. Being cheesed-off with him must burn calories, too.

No sex please, we're British

I believe that women and men have a fundamentally different attitude to sex after children. Women make love with their heads while men, well, we all know about that. What I mean is, that women have to be in the mood. They generally have to be schmoozed into it or slightly sozzled. Men are up for it at almost anytime of the day or night and anywhere in between. Women can go off sex for all sorts of reasons and they don't have to be logical ones at that – we might not have voiced a grudge, but our lack of interest in sex can voice this for us. Or is it that we are punishing our partners for getting us up the duff in the first place and a fear of this happening again is stopping the free flow of amour. This fundamental difference in attitude is quite confusing for everyone.

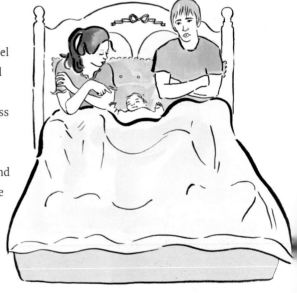

A bloke needs sex to feel he is being a real bloke and show his caveman-like prowess. It is good for stress relief and makes him feel close to you physically, mentally and spiritually. And you, you have to feel secure that this is love and not sex, that you are protected. Does something weird go on after becoming a mother, too? Somehow being a mother makes us think that we have responsibilities and that we haven't got that filthy hussy abandon that we had before motherhood.

If you are feeling that you would rather mop up the baby's poo than have sex, you are not alone. Sex is the glue that ultimately holds your relationship together, so getting down to it one day might be important. Don't despair – even bad sex is better than no sex. Check out these three great books that are worth a look at if you want to delve into this area further:

Baby-proofing your Marriage by Stacie Cockrell, Cathy O'Neill and
    Julia Stone (HarperCollins)
The New Mum's Guide to Sex by Rachel Foux (Fusion Press)
The Yummy Mummy's Survival Guide by Liz Fraser (HarperCollins)

On a practical note, obstetrician Dr Donald Gibb of the Birth Company (just in case you are planning any more) says that technically it is safe to have sex three weeks after birth as long as there are no stitches or you have not had a Caesarean. But more to the point, your head space has to be in the right place – and this might be more of a challenge than having your body in the right physical space.

Lucy's pelvic floor muscles really come into their own in this area girls – so get working! Well at least it's a start.

Be nice to yourself

* Don't worry if you don't feel up for it – it is normal.
* Remember that your partner has feelings too and sex is important to him – so work it out.
* Don't get a nubile au pair into your household before you've worked it out!

Body image

If you are a woman who hasn't been funny with food, then you are either lying or very lucky. Most of us have obsessed at various degrees of intensity from does my bum look big in this to full-blown problems of the serious or semi-serious kind. How we think we come across to others is vital as to how we handle our body perception. Yes, we might be overweight now (a baby has just hatched for pity's sake), but we can see this is not permanent and if we put the work in, all will not be lost or, to put it another way, all will be lost? We too often project forward to a place where we should be a size 10 and into our skinny jeans and in doing that we are confronted with the blinding truth – right now, we are Mrs Blimp and with no immediate prospect of getting the skinny jeans halfway up our thighs, let alone into an outfit combo. At that moment we think, 'Sod it! We'll never get there anyway, it's too depressing. A chocolate bar is the only thing that understands me.' Of course, one chocolate bar doesn't really do the damage, but an everyday chocolate bar habit soon adds up across a week.

Remember that you are beautiful just as you are. It is only you who says you are not. Your partner thinks you are beautiful. Blokes *hate* perpetual dieters. When you look in the mirror – and don't spend hours doing this or it will depress you, no matter how much you look like Kate Moss – look for the greatness in you. Look for the great teeth, gorgeous hair, nice hands, elegantly turned ankle, the Mona Lisa smile that plays across your cupid lips. Look for anything positive and don't focus on your butt or your stomach – most likely these are not your good features just now. They will be, but just now – as you are a normal woman – they might be a little compromised.

So love yourself *now* and if you really think you have a problem adjusting to Mrs Blimp then get some help to get your body image readjusted to the reality of now. It will get better and day by day you will be getting nearer to your goals.

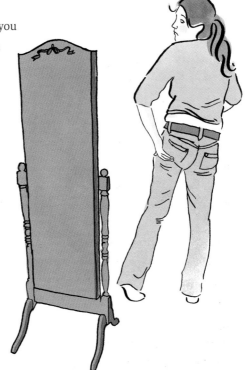

Be nice to yourself

✳ Love what you are *now* – love handles and everything.

✳ Focus on your good points and *not* on the negative ones – we can all find them once we start.

✳ Get hold of some serious dosh and hire an army of personal assistants to get you back in shape.

Good and bad — angel and devil

You know how it goes - you start
a new regime full of gusto and
after a couple of hours of really
sticking to the bright dawn of a new
beginning, you are patting yourself on
the back in a congratulatory kind of way.
Wow, you managed one whole day of
being *good* and after a week of adhering to the
programme, the halo has definitely been off for
a polish. My word, your fluffy angel wings of
righteousness are positively Persil white, with a
warm glowing goodess and purity. You have even
been tut-tutting a few of your friends lately for their
poor lifestyle and general slack exercise habits. And
their nutrition ... really! You've generally been giving
them the benefit of your new wisdom and conversion to
The Way.

Listen, you tell yourself with a small, knowing smile, you've
been so good, surely by now you deserve a little treat-ette? A
small, tiny gift to yourself just to reward all this good behaviour,
as a thank you. And anyway, if you don't give yourself a little
something now, you will cave in because you have been trying so
hard. Well, if you are going to have a little treat, you might as well
make it a good one. A giant icing-encrusted cream bun with all
the extras, including the cherry on the top.

And then it starts. The *bad*. Before you can say fire and
brimstone. Poof! A naughty little horned mini-you jumps on your

other shoulder. Look, you've had the bun, why not go for the pavlova and the chips too. Gooooo on! You know you want it. And you have been so perfect … how boring are you? Only real sissies and headgirl types are perfect. Now you don't have to be good any more, what damage can you cause? Hee hee! (evil chuckle).

When you've stopped your major *bad* fest, the beating yourself up stage follows – hair shirt and whip for extra effect (optional). Once you've gone down the cream bun route, what does it matter anyway? Might as well just go completely mad.

This sort of behaviour is normal when you start something new. The trick is not to judge food in terms of good or bad (or yourself, for that matter). You do the programme or you don't do the programme, but don't feel bad about it. Food is neutral. Only the choices are helpful or unhelpful depending on what you want to achieve (important reason for knowing what motivates you to get back into shape). Judging good and bad is like an elastic band being stretched back and back and sooner or later the band will snap the other way.

* Watch your language – how many times do you catch yourself saying either, 'I've been really good today' or, 'I had a terribly bad day'. Stop that. It's bad for your health.
* Don't judge food or yourself as good or bad – it won't help you in the long run.

Acting as if . . .

You have probably noticed one thing about being a mum. You spend an awful lot of time crawling round on your hands and knees. The ruin of many a good pair of trousers. Ever wondered where those dry patches on your knees came from? And no amount of any kind of exfoliating scrub gets rid of it in my experience. You don't have to look like Claudia Schiffer all the time. Indeed, it's impossible, but remember that how you look even to yourself and your baby is incredibly important because when you feel good you look good, and when you look good you feel great! So, however tempting it is to roam around the plains of your house with those giant tracksuit bottoms on, don't go there. You don't have Claudia's army of helpers, but looking half decent is a beginning – you are a mum, not Mr Blobby.

'Acting as if' is all about acting as if you *are* even if you are not, just now. You will be there faster by pretending you are already. With me so far? If you still feel like Mr Blobby, don't act it or you really will become Mr Blobby faster than you can say 'active waistband'. Apparently, the explosion of the leisure clothes market has had an equally explosive effect on our own waistbands. If we feel tightness around our girths, we apparently adjust our portion sizes downwards, but as stretch pants have no such control, we just go on eating. We don't know where the boundary is. Whatever you do, and however comfortable they may seem, junk those pants. Pretend you are feeling fabulous *now* and not slightly uncomfortable and super wobbly.

The expression 'it is what it is' is designed to make me see red, blue and purple because, of course, you can change what *it* is to something different and far brighter if you want to. You only have to know what that is and make a plan for a whole new incarnation. You are in the present moment and your starting point is now. That may be just exactly where you don't want to be, but the reality is you've had a baby, you've put on a few pounds and there is nothing you can do to make that picture different in the next five minutes. Now, if you take action, you can make that a different picture in the next five days, weeks, months and years, but right now it's a reality, so get used to it.

The only thing you can do at this point is pretend that it isn't as bad as you think and most often it really isn't as we are our own worst critics. Like the showman who carries on despite the worst, you must do the same. Look at really huge people who still look great even though they may not feel great inside. But I bet, like you, they don't look great without their make-up on. And unless you are very young with wonderful skin, neither will you.

Put on your face paint every day, even at home. With a tiny baby, you will have time when he is sleeping. With older children, it becomes a slight challenge as tiny hands are stuffed down your lipstick tube or your foundation erupts over everything. Whatever happens, persist with trying to look beautiful. You will be really glad you did.

Be nice to yourself

* You might not feel great, but pretend you do.
* You are where you are – no amount of wishful thinking is going to change that in the next five minutes.
* Put your make-up on every day – present a brave, can-do face to yourself and the world and, who knows, you might start to believe it!

Swedish mother

How come it is possible at one hundred paces to spot foreign mums? Is it their effortless chic, the film star shades and not having snail trails of toddler snot down their jumpers? Is it the perfect make-up and the way they skillfully glide in and out of several European languages as they chat and laugh at the school gates? How do they have the time? Once you actually talk to them, they are really nice, too. Don't you just hate them?

The Swedes are the worst. They really are very charming and very down to earth. I took my courage in both hands and stopped a perfect example of gracious motherhood in the park the other day. Not only a shining example of how to get out of the house remembering the baby and the five-year-old, but she didn't appear to have had the baby very recently as she was incredibly slender, calm and unruffled. She appeared to be *enjoying* herself and not shouting at the five-year-old, not even a bit. Just ambling along in near perfect-ness, a little blue butterfly fluttering around her strawberry blonde locks, flitting in and out of the golden sunbeams. As you know, you do have to be careful these days not to be mistaken for a potential nutter, so rather than surreptitiously hiding behind a tree trying to peek into the pram to ascertain how old the infant was, I went for the direct approach and decided to ask her outright. 'Madam, how old is that infant?', whereupon she most probably did think I was a nutter. To her credit she didn't run.

It turned out that she had had the baby two weeks ago. Two weeks?! Surely some mistake. On closer inspection of said infant, he (it turned out) was indeed squished enough to be two weeks old. How did she manage to look so toned and slim – was she famous? She didn't seem to be famous. She didn't appear to have several huge minders in suits talking into Bluetooth mobiles. No, it turned out she was a 'normal' Swedish mother. It transpired that not only has she not really put on much extra weight in pregnancy but her Swedish friends hadn't either.

On quizzing her further, it turns out that in Sweden they don't generally have a lot of convenience foods and most food is cooked fresh from scratch. A lot of Swedes are into healthy eating and muesli was practically invented in Sweden, she told me. They think nothing of having fish for breakfast – which, of course, as we know is perfect for balancing your blood sugar. They really don't have confectionary, either. Not like we do in England, she told me. It also turns out that a lot of Swedes have a great attitude to exercise and like to take health-giving saunas. So they have a better outlook when it comes to health and fitness to start with? Well, she couldn't speak for the whole of Sweden but generally, to be blunt, yes. She said how shocked she was at the state of our glorious nation and our attitude to food. Even the baby food. It is easy to find baby food with fish in Sweden. Good for all those clever Swedish brains no doubt. No wonder this country is going to the dogs – I was warming up for a rant.

During this pregnancy she had kept up the exercise by going to the gym every day, walking everywhere and even going swimming, too. She said this was normal for her. She didn't make an extra effort. She hadn't had any cravings either, only once for fresh pineapple – hardly a sin. Once a new patient of mine came in saying that it was all she could do to stop herself stuffing her face with Kentucky Fried

Chicken every day, even parking illegally and not caring if she got a ticket or her car was towed away. Then, Gollum-like, she would devour her prize, not even stopping to get the wrapper off. Thank God we stopped her doing that one.

So it turns out that Swedes are just healthier anyway. They are into eating fresh, healthy food and doing moderate exercise. My observation is they also seem to have a healthier body attitude, too – not so obsessed with celebrity and having to be thin. Swedes! Don't you hate them?

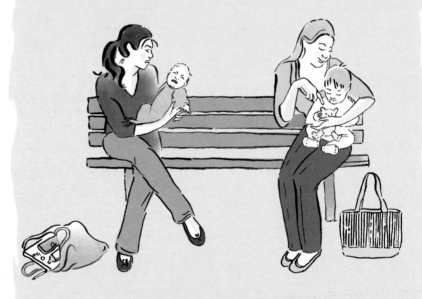

✳ It is easier to maintain your weight if you are Swedish –
   you will also be born with longer legs and naturally
   blonde hair – unfair, but true!
✳ Some cultures have healthier diets than us to start with,
   making it easier to maintain a healthier weight. We
   should try to learn a few lessons from them.

Difficulty shifting the weight

You know those people who say that they are overweight because they have a slow metabolism or because their parents were overweight or they only have to look at a cream bun to gain 400lbs? Well, what if one of those people is actually you? If you have done everything in this book, really put your back into it and the weight refuses to shift, then you might consider that something else is stopping you lose weight. Check out the following to see if any of the descriptions match your needs.

Emotional eating

* Do you lose weight and are really 'good' for ages only to scupper yourself at some point?
* Do you yo-yo diet?
* Do you reward yourself with food?
* Do you reach for the biscuit tin when you have had a 'bad' day?
* Do you eat when you are not hungry?
* Do you keep eating even if you are full?
* Do you consider that if you have eaten something that is not on the regime, that you have failed?

Solution: Consider going to hypnotherapy, counselling and improving self-esteem.

Obsessional or eating disorders

* Do you weigh yourself every day?
* Do you calorie count?
* Do you know how many calories are in a banana? (Trick question – if you do, you might be a walking calorie counter.)
* Have you tried every diet under the sun?
* Have you lied about when you last ate?
* Have you made yourself sick or tried laxatives?
* Have you ever got 'funny' about food?

Solution: There are specialist counsellors who deal in eating disorders, such as bulimia or anorexia.

Thyroid

* Are you constantly tired (silly question), but I mean really tired?
* Have you put on a lot more weight than you deserve plus are you finding it really difficult to shift?
* Are you constipated?
* Do you feel the cold?
* Do you have really dry skin?
* Are you depressed?
* Do you have shortened eyebrows?
* Are you losing hair, even six months after birth?

Your thyroid can often be challenged in pregnancy. The thyroid is a gland that has a few functions, but one of them is to help control your metabolism.

Solution: Go to see your GP and get a test for your thyroid. Check out a nutritional therapist in your area who could give you nutritional support.

Thrush or candida

* Do you have a white-coated tongue?
* Are you really tired?
* Have you put on loads more weight than you deserve and can't shift it?
* Are you prone to thrush?
* Are you prone to fungal infections, such as athlete's foot?
* Do you get bloating or gas after eating certain foods?

Some people are prone to being yeasty. If you are, it makes it really difficult to lose weight easily.

Solution: Find a nutritional therapist who can help you.

Hormone problems

* Are your periods regular?
* Do you suffer from PMS?
* Is the weight you are carrying on your hips and legs?
* Do you suffer from any female hormone condition such as endometriosis?

Disordered hormones can influence your weight.

Solution: Chinese herbal medicine (you need to have finished breastfeeding), nutritional therapy, exercise.

Adrenal problems (stress)

* Are you edgy and tense?
* Do you lose your temper over the slightest thing?
* Have you either lost your appetite or are eating for Britain?
* Do you normally carry extra weight around your middle?
* Are you sleeping badly (when you can sleep), or do you find it difficult to fall asleep?
* Are you a worry bug?
* Can you breathe without gasping for breath?

The stress hormone cortisol will encourage fat storage around your waist and you will be a typical apple shape.

Solution: Nutritional therapy, Chinese herbal medicine or acupuncture, exercise, relaxation, yoga.

Depression and anxiety

* Do you find it difficult getting up in the morning?
* Do you feel as if you are in a dark hole and can't get out, mood wise?
* Have you lost your sense of humour?
* Can't be bothered to look after yourself or to dress nicely?
* Can't be bothered to do anything?
* Have thoughts of harming either yourself or your baby?

Depression can prevent you wanting to do anything about your situation and makes you feel totally de-motivated.

Solution: Counselling, nutritional therapy (a nutrient deficiency could contribute to feeling low), exercise (yes, I know you can't be bothered, yet this is part of the solution for feeling better), connecting with other mothers. Having a baby can make you feel really out of control and sharing experiences can help.

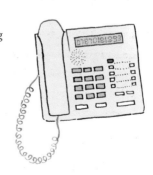

Supermodels and celebrity skinnies

How come it seems that three minutes after being released from the hospital, you see some gloriously elegant, svelte celeb saunter down an acreage of red carpet, flash bulbs a-popping looking like they've never been near a baby let alone just given birth to one?

I think it was Liz Hurley who admitted that she has to do the grind to look good, she has to actually try staying trim. Looking good from birth isn't something these people are born with, you know. You only have to remember Liz in *that dress* and take a peak through the safety pins that were holding it up to know that in those days she was quite a curvy girl, not at all the chiselled version we see in front of us today. Most celeb types realise only too keenly the cost equation between eating sausage and chocolate and their bank balances disappearing if they look anything less than perfect. And what an impossible gilded cage they lock themselves into, never being able to relax for a second, never gaining one pound without five million lenses eyeing them 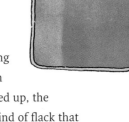 up and seeing exactly where that extra pound ended up, the speculation, the hype. You only have to read the kind of flack that Britney Spears got on account of a major junk food fest (and a major losing the plot episode), to know, when things go the other way, just how cruel and unforgiving the press can be.

Some celebs are so skinny they look like their head is about five times too big for their bodies – a broomstick with a pumpkin on top – not a good look. You know who you are. Also these super-skinny folk never look relaxed, at ease or happy with life. Instead they look super-stressed out and grumpy.

We really love those celebs who look real. Kate Winslet was furious when her legs were air brushed thinner for a cover shot of a men's mag – Kate is curvy, with great skin and a seemingly good attitude to both herself and food. A lifetime of being a pumpkin head comes at a cost. You cannot have one extra lettuce leaf without it popping out of your trousers somewhere.

So girls, no bashing yourselves up here. These guys have armies of staff to make it easy to ping back to their old shape – cooks and bottlewashers and a few personal trainers, nutritionists, stylists thrown in – you name it. We would all find it much easier to be supported in our mission 24/7 but, hey-ho, back to reality. If you are lucky enough to have help, use it and don't feel guilty and if you don't, well, it's much more satisfying doing it all by yourself anyway.

Be nice to yourself

* Invest in a software program with airbrush facility.
* Laugh at pumpkin heads.
* Embrace clever dressing.

Water retention

The hormonal changes that made you retain water in pregnancy struggle back to normal after birth and eating excessive amounts of food with sodium in it can encourage your body to hold on to fluid in the body. Bacon, crisps, canned and processed foods are not health products, so cut them out and in their place up the amount of potassium-rich foods. Loads of fresh fruit and veg will help counterbalance excessive sodium.

By the way, drinking loads of water, in a counter-intuitive way, actually helps flush out the system. Perhaps I should take this opportunity to remind you how much water you should drink a day: at least 1.5 litres (2½–3½ pints or about eight glasses). Get the glass you normally drink from and measure how much 1.5 litres actually is. You might

What body shape are you?
Moss, Madonna or Monroe

Good News! Your body shape is all pre-determined for you by your genes and hormones. Of course, this may not be such good news as you can't grow giraffe legs or become taller, but you can make the most of what nature has given you.

The Boffins have defined three major categories of body shapes – ectomorph, mesomorph and endomorph – so read on.

Moss

Although ectomorph sounds like some sort of an ectoplasmic encounter it is actually the body type that most defines the likes of Kate Moss – tall (OK, not for a supermodel, but she is quite tall compared to the rest of us), slim and with a small frame best describes this body shape. These types are often able to eat what they like without counting a single calorie or without the effort of trying to work off extra poundage by pounding frantically down the treadmill conveyor belt at the gym. This makes them far more interesting people, too – because of their natural thin genes, you'll never hear them moan about their weight or have to reassure them that they don't look fat in their skinny jeans. The ectomorph benefits from a genuinely fast metabolism and the best exercise for them is to strengthen the muscle and bones – and as these beanpole types tend to stoop, it's best to work on posture too. Shoulders back, stand tall. That's it.

Madonna

The mesomorph is of average height and tends to be more muscular (or a lot more muscular in Madonna's case – she has worked hard on those biceps to be fair to the rest of us). But watch it Madge, the abdominals can be an area where fat is easily stored. So if you are a mesomorph, putting in a bit of extra work on your abdominal training and power walking helps maintain a healthy weight – not something that Mrs Ritchie worries about, of course (I am sure she has masses of help with the diet from chefs, etc. and, boy, is she disciplined).

Monroe

The endomorph is that sexy, curvy, hourglass Monroe figure that stops men dead in their tracks with their tongues lolling out. Despite all these super skinny girls these days, many men like a little flesh on the bone. These types tend to store weight easily on the bottom, thighs and hips, a 'moment on the lips a lifetime on the hips' is the mantra of the Monroe types. Power walking is best for you. And so you don't get out of proportion, remember upper body training is key too.

Quick test

A way of telling what body type you are is to encircle your wrist with your thumb and middle finger. If your middle finger overlaps your thumb, then you are most likely to be an ectomorph. If your middle finger and thumb just touch, you are probably a mesomorph and if your finger and thumb do not touch, then you are most likely to be an endomorph.

Be nice to yourself

* Change your body type by cutting out a photo of your head and sticking it on a photo of Kate Moss's body.
* If you are the Marylin Monroe type, don't scoff too many cream buns – they will attach themselves to your hips (but at least you have a genuine excuse to say you have a slow metabolism).
* Make the most of your body type – it's here to stay.

find that you're struggling with big, huge glasses and don't need to drink eight of them!

If you are constipated, get it sorted as this is a major way to eliminate toxins. Oh, and the exercise thing actually helps fluid retention because it helps the lymph system move and the lymph system gets rid of toxins.

Be nice to yourself

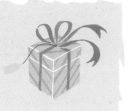

* Drink water.
* Take exercise.
* Eat lots of fresh fruit and veg.

The dreaded cellulite

Did you used to laugh at the Summer reports of those celebs with cellulite? 'Ha!,' you scoffed, 'there is no way my legs will ever look like a giant orange.' How wrong you were. Fear not:

* First of all, eating a healthier diet will help, including loads of fruit and veg.
* Us nutritional therapists think that if the load on your liver is reduced (not so many hormones whizzing around), that will be helpful. So now you are not pregnant that might help somewhat.
* Drink loads of water.
* Get that body brush out that is lurking in the bottom of your bathroom cupboard and get brushing. Use upward strokes on the thighs and stomach, but don't be too hard on yourself, body brushes can be quite brutal (*see* opposite).
* Mix together 12 drops of grapefruit pure essential oil, 10 drops of juniper pure essential oil and 2 tablespoons of sweet almond oil and massage on to your dodgy bits.

A collection of body brushes and what do with them

At the last count I had at least four body (completely new) brushes. The trick is to actually put them to good use and not just collect them, squirreling them along with the small shop's worth of beauty products, potions and other fads in your bathroom cupboard. Lucy has persuaded me to start using one of mine – the one with the long handle – but be careful. I actually, and I am yet to know how, hit myself between the eyes when the head of the brush flew off across the room and ricocheted off the wall, finding its target.

Body brushing helps our lymphatic drainage system to remove toxins from the body and in doing so is said to reduce cellulite in our thighs and bottom where fats, proteins and other waste products tends to accumulate. If you

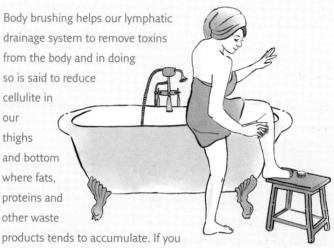

do this twice a week before you step into the bath or shower when the body and the brush are dry, not only do you feel invigorated but in a short time you begin to look fab, too.

Start brushing from your feet, brushing in long strokes up your legs and then towards the groin, work in circular motions over your tummy (gently). Then do your arms, shoulders and chest. Your skin may redden and start tingling because the brushing increases the circulation in areas where there is more fat accumulation.

Home spa or spa treat

If you feel you are taking care of yourself on the outside, then pretty soon you will feel that this begins to reflect on the inside, too. I promise. Feeling that you are worth it is extremely important to help you maintain a positive outlook on life and boost your self-esteem and everyday confidence. If you are feeling all grey and sluggish and the hair on your legs is enough to knit a scarf with, you need to do something urgently. It may all seem to be horribly self-indulgent to pamper yourself, but you are doing this for the world – your own little world anyway. A grumpy, depressed mum with hairy armpits is no good to anyone. In order for your family to be happy, you need to be happy and glorious first.

The very best thing to do, of course, is to take some time out, get in a baby-sitter and cruise out to the local day spa. Number one priority is the de-fuzz. There is nothing more depressing than black hairy legs poking out below your sweatpants. The next step (and this is a good cheap way to lift the years and the cares away from your face) is to have a professional eyebrow shape. Look carefully at the therapist's own first – no eyebrows or eyebrows drawn in with a pencil is a really bad sign. Run for the hills.

Then give yourself a delicious treat. A facial is always great because, realistically, it is something that you may never do yourself. Also, they sometimes do stuff that frankly you are not interested in doing or don't feel you have the time for, like a treatment mask. Massages are always great, too. If you don't know much about

Stretchmarks

It's best to try to prevent stretchmarks in the first place by making sure the skin is in super fantastic condition before getting pregnant. If that's all too late, try rubbing special oils enriched with all sorts of luscious goodies onto the skin – a good excuse to treat yourself. Or break open a couple of capsules of vitamin E and rub the contents into the stretchmarks.

Vitamins A, C and E and zinc are all good for skin health. They won't repair the damage, but we don't want any others forming, now, do we? Yet another reason for eating your greens and getting on the nutritional road.

Fitness for your face

Make sure that you get your partner to take the baby out for a long walk then give yourself time to give yourself an energising face lift – no messy, expensive surgery, no bruising or recovery time. Just good clean *fun!* And all these ingredients you can find in your very own kitchen – well almost all of them.

All you need is several drops of oil – almond oil for fair skin, olive for dark and jojoba for sensitive skin. Put eight drops into the palm of your hand and apply all over your face. Then apply your home-made facial exfoliative – two heaped teaspoons of fine oatmeal with several drops of whichever oil you choose, made into a paste. Using the pads of your fingers, rub it evenly over all your face and neck with a light action. Don't forget to rub a little of the mixture onto the lips to plump them up. Leave on for a few minutes then rinse off the mixture with warm water. This beauty mask removes any dead skin cells, improves your circulation and gives you super smooth skin.

massages, go for an intensive back and shoulder massage. I've never seen the point in them doing your legs and arms and all the turning over spoils the relaxation bit of it, too.

Not prepared to splash out the time or the money? Fear not. You can create your own home spa. The trick is not to not start because you think you won't have the time; just do a little each day. Start with a luxurious bath, even if that is in the baby's rest time in the middle of the day. Use as many oils and creams as you want. Moisturising, moisturising, moisturising is the key. Truly worthwhile products are never cheap, but think of all the money you are saving by staying at home.

Be nice to yourself

❋ Making yourself beautiful saves the world.
❋ Feeling great on the outside, makes you feel glowing on the inside – so do it.
❋ Don't feel guilty about taking time out for yourself – it is really hard work being a mum.
❋ Save money at the salon and buy in the stuff – this will work out cheaper, you hope.

Help yourself . . .

. . . by getting support

Making plans, making plans, don't you just love making plans? The thing about plans is that it is great to have them, but then you have to do something about what you have written down. A tonne of planning is worth an ounce of theory. We already know the first thing we have to do with a plan is to write it down – it doesn't have to be on a brand new pad with sharpened pencils – the back of an envelope would do just fine.

Shout from the rooftops

Who is going to help you make your plan a success? Declaring you have a plan is often a great way to make sure you stick to your intentions. Having your partner remind you that you have made a promise to yourself is a great way to actually make things happen. You'll do it to stop him nagging and to prove him wrong. Also you need his support as he will be your main source of delegating baby to when you need time to exercise or whatever.

A friend in need

What about getting another mum to swap baby-sitting time with? You could look after her baby and, of course, the plan would be that she would look after your baby for an afternoon a week. You could even get fit and healthy together.

A mum to lean on?

If you have a mum or mother-in-law nearby, you can always rope them in, too. Schedule in a regular time for them to visit, just as long as you don't have the kind of mum that wants to 'help' when really it feels more like she is criticising. If any sentence starts with, 'In my day,' you know it is not the kind of help or suggestion you want. Everyone who helps you in your mission of claiming back the old you should be 110 per cent supportive, or don't tell them what you are up to. It doesn't take long for an Eeyore attitude to bring your bright new shiny plan nose bombing to the floor. Who wants someone raining on your parade? Bright cheery, can-do folk is what you want.

Consider hiring help

We all know that money does not grow on trees, at least not in my neck of the woods, but sometimes it might be worth thinking about buying in some help, even for the short term.

Au pairs can be a great help with the daily chores and good company if you are on your own at home. Or they can be a complete disaster. They might just be a little too young and a little bit too attractive for your liking but not for your partner's; they may think they are speaking perfect English – and they are definitely talking very fluently – but the only slight snag is, you haven't a clue what they are on about; they might also give absolutely no notice of leaving and leave you high and dry or be so homesick that they never really settle in because they are trying to get home as often as they can (and with cheap flights these days that is entirely possible). Here, however, are some tips for making the au pair story a good one:

* Personal recommendation of a good agency is key – the agency will handle disasters.
* Do check out the references, but not via mobile numbers. If the reference is talking with an unbelievably thick accent, it is probably their mum.
* Make sure your au pair really does speak good English, or your child's first language could be exotic.
* Although it sounds quite draconian, make sure you have the house rules drawn up in writing as this will help avoid misunderstandings and then everyone knows where they stand.

Be nice to yourself

✳ Get your plan out in the open – telling others makes you more likely to succeed.

✳ Get the support of your other half, both emotionally and physically.

✳ Can you rope in another family member who might like to baby-sit?

✳ Could you afford to pay for some child cover, even for a couple of afternoons a week?

✳ Could you swap baby-sitting with another mum who wants to get fit?

✳ Join a gym with a crèche.

. . . to cope with a difficult baby

The worst thing for knocking you off the old nutritional and exercise horse is if events are taken out of your hands and, for all your trying, you find that you really can't control circumstances. Truly the most difficult of these blockers is if you have drawn the short straw on the crying baby. Well you'd hate to call him difficult, but in plain speech that is being polite, frankly. Whatever you do, however you do it, your baby will just not stop crying and, in fact, when you do try, the volume knob goes up a couple of notches instead of down. This can be unbelievably de-motivating, demoralising and just downright depressing.

Some babies pop out with a smile and all is right and bright with the world. That smug mother in playgroup who says her baby sleeps through the night (bet she is wearing ear plugs and has the monitor on silent). Of course, *her* baby eats everything and weaning was a cinch. Perfect, perfect, perfect. Other babies are plainly really cheesed off at having been yanked into the light and into reality, and are not happy bunnies at all. Sleep? You only have to be thinking of her, and by some unknown telepathic power, you have managed to wake her. Creeping into her room, despite tinkling on the tips of your toes and the siren goes up, 'WAAAAAA!', just as your mission is about to be accomplished.

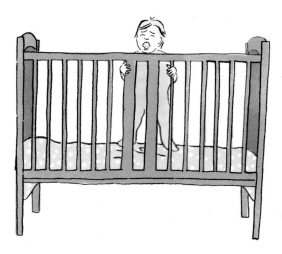

Cranial sacral osteopathy

If you are up for alternative solutions, you might want to try to take your infant to a cranial sacral osteopath. Go on a good recommendation ... any yummy mummy will point you in the right direction. As birth can be quite traumatic (just a bit), cranial oestopaths use very gentle techniques to help realign the head – I know it sounds weird, but babies can transform in good hands.

Homeopathy

Try a homeopath (again, a recommendation is essential). With homeopaths it either works in a spectacular way or doesn't work at all. Either way it is safe. You must have a good practitioner as homeopaths have to be skilled at working out which remedy is going to work. I personally am a huge fan.

Explore the windy route

Is wind a problem? Not for you, for the baby. Try adding some special friendly bacteria to feeds (if your baby takes a bottle) as this can rebalance and help his tiny gut. Of course, friendly bacteria added to formula is easy if you are entirely bottle feeding and, if this is your route, check that the formula is not causing the problem. Some babies have an easier time on goat's formula as the protein in goat's milk is easier to digest. The organic goat's milk brands also tend not to add a whole lot of other ingredients, such as sugar, to their products – you'd be surprised how much the quality varies in standard formula. Look for brands with not too much sugar (sugar is disguised as anything ending in '-ose'). If confused, have a chat with your nutritional therapist or your health visitor.

Washing powder

It may also be worth checking your washing powder. Some babies' skin is really sensitive and it can feel like there is an ant in their sleeping suit if the washing powder doesn't agree. Non-biological brands are less likely to cause this problem.

Of course, if you are really worried about why your baby is crying so much, maybe she is in pain. Check out any serious worries with your doctor.

Be nice to yourself

* Don't take crying babies personally – they do love you, really.
* Try to get out of the house. Get someone to look after him for an hour or you will go nuts.
* Check out what might be causing it and take some action – doing something will make you feel better.

... to continue running your own business

You decided to set up your own business so that you could be your own boss, take off time when you wanted, so that you could be more flexible and work less punishing hours, right? Wrong! Day one you realised you had made a *huge* mistake, *massive*. How you had imagined those sunny days, sitting sipping your cappuccino making executive calls on your mobile. Working on public holidays and not taking a proper break, more like! Before the baby forced you to take the time off, you worked harder than you have ever worked before because, when you have your own business, it is all down to you. You can't delegate that to the nerdy gnome in the IT department; you *are* the IT department. And as for that nightmare boss ...

Post baby, after parking your career and company for a while, it's time to get back in the driving seat but *time* ... oceans of glorious time have dried up before your very eyes and you are not in control of it like you were. How can you fit in running the business, exercising, nutrition and feeding the baby when you didn't even do any of these 'luxuries' when you did have the space? First day on your new exercise regime, all changed into your Lycra-stretch gear, little Johnny decides it is the first time he is going to projectile vomit everywhere – starting with your new exercise outfit and ending up all over the walls. That's the end of that then. At least 50 calories burnt changing outfits and a couple of hundred in cleaning the walls. Fabulous.

At first glance, the solution seems quite contradictory – be flexible and be a better planner of your time.

Be as flexible as possible

Flexiblity comes with not being really rigid with your thinking. Aim to say with a gracious smile that, 'This was meant to be,' and try not to kick the dog. Go with it. Beating yourself up isn't going to help and using it as an excuse not to ever exercise again is a bit self-defeating.

Plan your time

Planning your time is a way to prevent these curved balls of unfortunate events coming in and ruining everything. As an international businesswoman you are quite used to planning your time in a business environment, but your own time – well, that feels a little too much like obsessive-compulsive disorder. You are *creative* (swish hair and said with a flourish) and you don't have time to plan. Well, pal, you don't have time not to. When you run your own business, unlike in the magazines where 'effortlessly' and 'juggle' are words that are just lies made up by PR people, if you don't run your business, it will run you.

Time will be squeezed if you don't plan it. It will be taken away from somewhere and usually this is family time – family don't normally shout as loud as your most demanding customer. This must be some law of physics, but us business owners just try to fit the pint pot in the quart jar of time, like a mad magician. Instead of being in control, all you are is mega stressed-out.

Planning your time can be a daunting prospect but if you want to get back to the trim, healthy, happening old you, then planning is your only option. All the good intention in the world is not going to make you exercise or take care of your nutrition. When you run your own business, you are the last priority. Ever noticed that? And now that you have your baby to care for, well it's even more important that you take control (*see* The eight-step guide to getting under control, overleaf).

Be nice to yourself

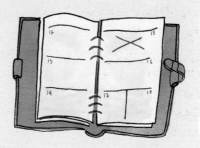

* Prioritise your home-time first, then fit in the rest of your tasks.
* Plan your time with a strategy calendar and plan to make exercise and nutrition happen.
* Get proper childcare help so that you are not trying to keep one eye on the baby, one eye on the emails, another on the phone – not an efficient way to keep your busy working life on track.
* Get a student to help you with your admin.
* Book exercise time in the diary and don't let yourself down by moving it out – easy to do when you have demanding clients. Give yourself permission to take this important time off for your own health, sanity and self-esteem.
* Allow more time than you think exercising will need – plan for success.
* Be flexible. When all the good planning turns to filth, go with the flow.
* Don't feel guilty.

The eight-step guide to getting under control

1 Get a blank piece of paper and put at the top 'Annual strategy'. What do you want to achieve with your business this year? Write it down.

2 Make a heading, 'Quarterly strategy'. What do you need to do this quarter to get to the annual strategy?

3 Work out what your monthly strategies would have to be to achieve your quarterly goals.

4 Get a calendar page for the month and allot time to the tasks that are going to get you to your goals.

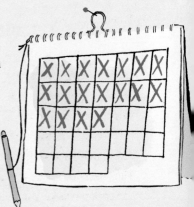

5 With the business strategy taken care of, you can afford to now allow time for your personal goals. Imagine that your time is like a jar and in that jar you have put some big rocks, which represent the important, immovable stuff – your exercise and nutrition. On your strategy calendar, first block out the time you need to achieve this. Be generous. There is nothing worse than having all these great plans, ideas and intentions and then feeling really frustrated as week after week disappears in little puffs of smoke. You will just end up feeling totally inept.

6   Add the gravel, which represents the other stuff – work, meetings – and finally the sand – these are all the little irritating things you have to do like emails and phone calls. Be disciplined with emails. Only check them twice a day. Remember that someone else's *urgent* isn't necessarily your urgent. Let them wait. If you are not careful, your life and intentions and your goals are pulled off course by other people's plans. Don't let this happen to you or your dream of being a yummy mummy will disappear as fast as you can say 'send/receive'.

7   Essential to your planning when building in exercise into your business life is getting a really good person you can delegate to, even when you run your business from home. In the end, although an expense, it might be worth it. Work out how much your time is actually worth in money terms and it might be a real eye opener to see that masses of it is gobbled up with admin and 'sand' tasks. University students need the dosh – not like the good old days when the State paid for everything. They need jobs. Doing your admin is arguably a lot better than working in Maccie D's. You could argue that one certainly.

8   On a Sunday night, scope out your week. Block out your rocks, gravel and sand time and make a list of everything you have to do for the week ahead. Give it a specific time in your diary. When can you do it? Once there, it will get done.

. . . by chunking it down

Don't you absolutely hate people who say, 'If you want to eat an elephant, use a teaspoon'? Annoying, but absolutely true. Even more annoying when it is true, don't you find? Of course, eating an elephant with a teaspoon means that if a project is too whoppingly big, don't look at the entire thing, chunk it down. Chunk it down into very small bits and if you keep going long enough, you will eventually have achieved your aim.

We tend to globalise our goals into a huge great mountain to climb, which seems so impossible it is tempting not to start at all. At the moment you might feel like your body has been hi-jacked by aliens or that you have borrowed a fat suit from a movie prop department and, yes, it is a good idea to have an idea of the big thing you want to achieve to inspire you, but not at the expense of depressing yourself. If you are not fit now, you will be. But accept you are not fit just now. Don't give up right at the beginning. Of course you are not fit now, but that's why you are making all this effort, isn't it? You may feel like you can't do a press-up (even the really easy ones), well never mind. Who is judging you except yourself? Going round the park at a very slow, graceful plod, seems like it is doing nothing – and especially if you are not really feeling it. But it is working, I promise you. Any exercise and any improved nutrition will work as long as you just do a little of it every day.

So get your big goal or compelling vision and chunk it down. If your ambition is to get into a size 12, make it a 14 first. Don't be perfect, just be better. If you want to run the marathon, make it a 10km (6 mile) 'moon walk' first, then plan for the big one.

Measure your progress with marker posts. Aim at first for five circuits around the park and then go for the ten sprint versions when you are up to it. Just keep going. Don't give up. You are never quitting as long as you are still in the game of trying. However many times you start and 'fail', if you are still up for trying, you are going to get there in the end.

Be nice to yourself

* Eat a *huge* chocolate ice cream elephant with a teaspoon (yes, you heard it here first folks).
* Chunk down your goals – and make sure you know when you are making progress by setting reasonable targets.
* Don't look back and regret how you were (or have fantasies about being Kate Moss), look to today. A great today leads to better tomorrows.

. . . by creating a compelling vision

Compelling vision – what does that mean? It means, girls, that when you start a new programme or project, you have to be really up for it or it just won't happen. You have to know where you are going. You have to know what the end is going to look like or you will have no inspiration as to why you might turn down that extra chocolate biscuit. How often have we all said, 'Monday, latest Tuesday, I am going to get my act together,' and then not done a blind thing about it? Of course, we mean it at the time, but other things get in the way, don't they? Like shopping, and going out to lunch, a glass of wine – and, frankly, they are much more exciting than any perceived restrictions and deprivations. Who wants the prospect of cardboard biscuits with cottage cheese? Next week suddenly gets all the promises – and, of course, next week never, ever comes.

So, compelling vision is the reason why you might put yourself to an extra amount of work. A bit more exercise, cooking and nutrition. All this with a baby to contend with. Why put yourself through all that extra effort? Compelling vision, that's what. So, a compelling vision is a picture in your head of what it would be like to have achieved your perfect weight. Remember too, that there is no such thing as perfect – it is only perfect for you. Don't be guided by 'shoulds' or what other people look like – perfect is *your* perfect and no one elses.

Furthermore, this compelling vision doesn't have to be a great big thing, it can be a small thing. Whatever inspires you. But it helps if you have a picture of what this looks like in your head. It also really helps if you put it down on a piece of paper somewhere, even if you never look at it again. I have a lady who comes to see me who wants to wear an aquamarine swimming costume next summer and be able to have the soft, lolling waters of the Med wash gently over her as she lies on her tummy at the shore-line, listening to the breath of the sea sighing sweetly. Not much to ask? For her this is *huge* – she hasn't been swimming for years – and in a swimming costume with everyone watching, she's understandably frightened. But she'll do it. This image inspires her and motivates her to keep to the programme, even when the chocolate and cream buns hone into view.

Too tired to exercise? Can you do it if you have something to inspire you? Inspiration will be unique to you – a 10km (6 mile) race, for example, or do you want to be lithe enough to play with your kids? Get that vision there in your head, ladies, and you can achieve anything.

Be nice to yourself

- Start with the end in mind – a picture to inspire you when the going gets tough.
- Write it down, even if you never look at it again.
- Just because some of these supermodels look like a broomstick with a pumpkin on the top doesn't mean that you have to as well.

... by considering hypnotherapy

You are determined to lose weight and you are getting on fabulously, but just when you think you are getting somewhere, the call of the biscuit tin is just too loud and all that hard work turns to dust as you pile back the pounds. You know what to do, it's just that some mysterious power is too great. Perhaps it's time to consider hypnotherapy?

When I have my clinician's hat on and I am working with new mums in my clinic, I approach getting back into shape not only from the nutrition point of view but from an holistic perspective, too. I want new mums to feel confident, inspired, energetic and to overcome some of the seemingly insuperable barriers that can scupper best-intentioned efforts. I have a bank of other experts who help me do this. David Samson is one important part of the team that I call on. David is a hypnotherapist, who 'unknots' the unknown reasons of why we get stuck in the same old, sometimes destructive, habits. Every case history is different, but in a way Sophie is typical.

Sophie's choice — biscuits

Nine months after the birth of her first child, Sophie was still struggling to lose the extra pounds gained during her pregnancy. She had tried all the traditional dieting methods but appeared to have a 'mental block' that prevented her from shaking off those pounds. She always started a new regime with gusto, but rapidly lost this enthusiasm and sneaked back to her old habits.

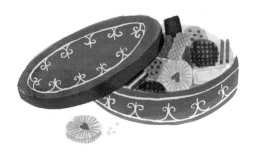

During her initial meeting with David a few clues began to emerge to explain this pattern of yo-yo dieting. Sophie's husband was still ecstatic about the birth of his daughter and constantly praised Sophie for giving him 'the best present in the world'. Sophie's mother also regularly complimented her. The more compliments she received, the more rapidly her dieting attempts seemed to fail. On the surface, Sophie appeared to be an emotional eater with links between praise and reward, but her subconscious mind would reveal the extent of this issue while under hypnosis.

There are two basic hypnotherapy techniques – the one you see on TV is called 'suggestion' hypnosis where the hypnotist makes suggestions to the person in trance.

The second technique, favoured by David, is called 'regression' hypnotherapy where the hypnotised person remembers childhood incidents and reinterprets them as an adult and can subsequently make a permanent change to a particular behaviour.

In Sophie's case, the reasons for her inability to lose weight became obvious pretty quickly to David. During their second session, she remembered a scene as a three-year-old. She was sitting on her mother's lap learning to read. Her mother was extremely loving and very generous with her cuddles. However, her mother had learned something from her own mother that she subsequently passed on to Sophie ... there was a link between food and love. While in hypnosis, Sophie remembered her mother's praising words as she hugged her, 'you are my special girl, you read that page all on your own and now I'm going to bake you some fairy cakes.' As a three-year-old, the link had been confirmed – if you do something well, you get a cuddle and some nice food.

During subsequent sessions, this link that had been learnt at such a young age was confirmed with a number of events that Sophie remembered in which she was rewarded for her achievements with food.

This visit into the past allowed Sophie to realise that she was continuing to follow the same pattern in the present day. Her husband's praising sent her rushing for the cookie jar to reward herself for producing such a fine baby. Her genuine attempts to lose weight were being thwarted by her subconscious, which was thriving on the food/love/reward connection.

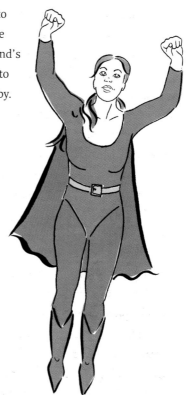

This realisation caused a major change in her eating habits, but Sophie now fully understands her previous behaviour and her reactions to praise. She has settled into a healthy eating and exercise pattern and her weight is falling off quite naturally. She is now looking forward to a lifetime of happiness with her new family with plenty of cuddles ... but no cookies!

Be nice to yourself

✴ There is no shame in getting help if you need it.

✴ Get a good recommendation from a friend – the best way to find someone good who you can trust.

Struggling mum

Rachel is really keen to lose the baby weight she has put on with the beautifully big-eyed, lovely natured Samantha. Rachel is absolutely beautiful if only she would see it! She has dark flowing hair, lovely skin. She is half Italian, which gives her a charming lilt to her voice and an attractive turn of phrase. Of course, having the Italian influence really works to her advantage on how she dresses too – elegant and understated. Rachel glides across a room. She is tall, so she really 'holds' the room.

Rachel has never been one for formal exercise, but she is prepared to walk and do outside stuff although with a newish baby (nine months) she never seems to find the time. She has grasped the principles of the eating plan with gusto – she really gets it. On her last visit she made wonderful progress and really started to get back to getting trim. She had lost a whole lot of poundage from her mid-rift and she was really happy with her progress. A month later, though, and she is back where she started and feeling very low about her progress. What started as a little chocolate treat has developed in to a full blown chocolate habit and all in a month. The biscuit tin beckoned, too. One biscuit is never really enough, is it?

We chat about her background. It turns out that her mum was always on a diet herself and when she was growing up in exotic China, they never had biscuits or sweets in the house and to have something 'naughty' was a reward for good behaviour. Her mother was really disciplined with her diet and wouldn't allow herself to go off-beam without a real fight with herself.

Rachel might be the ideal candidate to look into hypnotherapy. I know it sounds really spooky and that someone is messing with your head, but professional hypnotherapists are not like the ones you see on the TV that are going to turn you into Elvis Presley or make you walk around like a chicken. Our subconscious minds are where we store a lot of our early programming that comes from our early childhood. From birth to about seven years old we are very susceptible to the influence of everything around us – a lot of our messages, of course, come from our parents and their attitudes, but even seemingly innocuous comments can be grabbed by the subconscious mind and then run as our operating programme for the rest of our lives. You can change this programming by being conscious – knowing that you are influenced by your childhood – or get professional help to prompt change.

My advice to Rachel

* First, don't judge happiness on the scales – we all have times where we are on the programme and times when the whole thing turns to filth, so don't judge yourself in the dip.
* Love yourself *now* – don't wait.
* If it all goes horribly wrong, start again by just getting breakfast 'right'. Don't try to climb the mountain of trying to do everything perfectly.

. . . to understand breastfeeding better

You know what they say? 'Breast is best.' You know this by now or you have been living on planet Zog, but don't feel guilty if the breastfeeding bit is not happening for whatever reason (incompatible nipples; too tired and milk stops; you can't because you are taking medication). In the Sixties and Seventies it all became a bit socially unacceptable for mothers to breastfeed and it was thought that the bottle was a lot more dignified and probably a lot more convenient too, as you could then delegate childcare, thus allowing the Sixties' hippy mother to go off to a peace camp, smoke drugs or make more babies - whatever hippies got up to in the Sixties.

Anyway, the point is it can be difficult and not necessarily the ideal of that snugly one-to-one moment of bonding merrily. Of course, if it all works out well, it is lovely to have that tiny bean staring into your eyes with an expression of true love. Nothing like it.

Breastfeeding is obviously convenient. None of that sterilising the bottles nonsense or packing up a huge bag of spare bottles when you go away and the milk is pre-warmed and full of the right vitamins and minerals for your baby's health. It also has the *big* advantage of pulling in the uterus. This means that all the time when junior is sucking away, you are getting thinner without even trying *and* you are burning 500 extra calories a day.

But the downside is that you can't share the night shift (well, any shift) with your partner and it can be a lonely old time getting up at 3am with nothing but the moon, the Bean and an owl for company.

The pros of breastfeeding

* Breastfed babies get a head start as breast milk has high levels of DHA (fat), which is good for the brain.
* The milk is easily absorbed so is better for all-round health.
* There are lots of minerals in breast milk – selenium, for example – that is not in formula.
* Breast milk helps establish a good gut colony of friendly bacteria for the baby's gut.

The cons of breastfeeding

* Your partner can't do the night shift.
* It can be knackering, especially after a difficult birth where you take longer to recover anyway.
* You have to make sure you are having a good diet to help overcome the tiredness – the breast milk's quality will suffer if you are under the weather.

If you are breastfeeding

* Drink enough water – you need loads – or the milk can be difficult to produce. You need to aim for as much as 3 litres (5 pints), which I appreciate is difficult when you are racing around and adjusting to a new way of life, but it will help make the whole process so much easier.
* Eat enough. If you are not eating enough, the weight will fall off too quickly and you will just end up feeling very tired. But don't be tempted to pile into the cream buns, instead get extra calories from:

- Eating bigger portions.
- Eating fives times a day (breakfast, lunch and dinner and two snacks).
- Eating food with lots of healthy oils – like avocado, oily fish – and plenty of good carbs like brown rice, sweet potatoes and whole grains (millet, barley, rye and spelt, are examples).
- Taking vitamins and minerals. You need loads of zinc – the baby needs about 3mg per day and most often there is not enough zinc in the breast milk. Of course, eat more zinc foods like chicken, lamb, turkey, nuts and seeds, but in the end it might be quicker to supplement it with a good multi-vitamin (*see* page 69). Zinc is good for your immune system so, if you are not getting enough, you can get very run down if you are breastfeeding for a long time. If you are using formula for your baby, make sure it has plenty of zinc, B vitamins and an essential fatty acid.

Another part of the A-team

My colleague and friend Catriona Muir, is a lovely midwife who you would definitely want looking after you during the birth of your baby and preferably for the rest of your life, too. She is one of those people who inspire masses of confidence, which is something that new mums sometimes lack when it comes to breastfeeding. Catriona is someone I turn to if I have a mum who can't cope with feeding a new baby with her own God-given equipment.

As a midwife, Catriona spends much time with women during the ante- and postnatal periods discussing breastfeeding. Midwives have a professional responsibility to encourage best practice and to ensure that women are given appropriate, accurate and unbiased information to allow them to make fully informed decisions. During the Sixties and Seventies, people began to get quite prudish about breasts and breastfeeding in general (I know, quite a few young people at the time were busy showing their breasts to all and sundry but the Establishment – *they* were quite tut, tut about boobs). Anyway, there's a theory coming up, I am not sure about this, but perhaps with the advent of such grown-up products as Bird's Custard and Cadbury's Smash – 'they' (the people who decide these things) thought they could do a whole lot better than nature with a tin of powder and a bit of water. As a result, many of today's mums didn't breastfeed their babies to be able to teach their daughters. The long and short is that many mothers lack confidence in their ability to breastfeed their baby today. Catriona tells me that in many cases this is aggravated by a similar lack of confidence among their partners. When she asks a new mother how she plans to feed her baby, it is quite common to hear, 'Well I'd like to give it a go,' rather than it being a given that she *is* going to breastfeed the baby.

Catriona says that although most women are aware of at least some of the benefits of breastfeeding, many assume that they will run into problems such as not having enough milk or have concerns about the size and shape of their breasts and/or nipples. Breasts and nipples come in all different sizes and shape and it is reassuring to know that all are suitable for breastfeeding. Yes folks, you heard it here first. Sometimes, however, the size and shape of the nipple may mean that mother and baby need particular help to achieve effective attachment and success. If this sounds like you, you need someone like Catriona to show you how it is done. Once mastered, very few women actually can't breastfeed.

Benefits for the mother – some surprising information

There is increasing evidence of long-term health benefits from breastfeeding for the mother. These include:

* Breastfeeding plays a natural part in helping mothers to lose the extra weight gained during pregnancy.
* A reduction in the incidence of pre-menopausal (and possibly post-menopausal) breast cancer, and some forms of ovarian cancer.
* A lower incidence of hip fractures in women over the age of 65.
* A delay in the return of fertility.

Midwife Catriona's benefits of breastfeeding

Breastfeeding has a long-term role in child health. Moreover, breastfeeding helps to protect a mother's health in several ways and can therefore benefit the whole family, emotionally and economically. Research has shown the following health outcomes for breastfed babies:

* Reduced incidence of gastrointestinal and respiratory infections during the neonatal period and later.
* Reduced incidence of glue ear.
* Reduced incidence of diabetes as a young child or adult.
* Better development, especially in preterm babies, of the brain, central nervous system and sight.
* Lower blood pressure in later childhood and possibly adulthood.
* Reduced incidence of wheezing during childhood.
* Reduced incidence of obesity, in both child- and adulthood.
* Reduced incidence of urinary tract infection.
* Improved response to immunisation.

There is increasing evidence of other important benefits to the baby:

* It is suggested that the incidence of some childhood cancers is reduced (lymphoma and Hodgkin's disease).
* Certain allergic conditions may be less severe.
* Some studies show a lower incidence of sudden infant deaths.
* There may be a reduced risk of developing multiple sclerosis.

Natural worries

Worries that Catriona comes across are varied but many mothers believe that they do not have enough milk or that their milk is 'too thin'. This is usually because their breasts do not seem to them to be full; because the milk appears watery; or because their baby's behaviour suggests that he is hungry. Sometimes it is some well-meaning member of the family who suspects that the quantity or quality of her milk is poor, which can affect a new mother's confidence in her ability to feed her baby properly. Just remember that you managed to grow this baby somehow – that's pretty amazingly clever. Man has got this far breastfeeding babies and there are an awful lot of us humans that prove the method is at least somewhat successful.

Another worry that Catriona comes across is the panic that mothers don't eat enough or aren't getting enough nutrients. If they try to get their shape back early, somehow they will be harming the baby. Here are more excuses to eat for two.

In reality, the stores of nutrients need to be extremely low before there is any significant impact on the nutritional qualities of breast milk and it is very rare for any of the diet to be deficient, at least in Britain. Remember that you do need extra calories (more food) whilst you are breastfeeding – about 500 calories more – but make a note to self: the cream buns aren't necessary – good nutritious food will do. Our expert Catriona says that you will not do yourself or the baby any harm by steadily working to getting your shape back while breastfeeding.

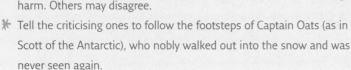

Be nice to yourself

✳ Relax – you can do it. And if you can't, you can't. Don't stress. I was bottle-fed and it never did me any harm. Others may disagree.

✳ Tell the criticising ones to follow the footsteps of Captain Oats (as in Scott of the Antarctic), who nobly walked out into the snow and was never seen again.

Some breastfeeding myths

The list of untrue statements on breastfeeding is staggering.
They are too numerous to mention here, but these are some of
the better known:

Myth 1: Breastfeeding ruins the shape of your breasts.
Reality: This is simply not true. As soon as a woman becomes
pregnant, permanent changes occur in her breasts. Whether or not
she then goes on to breastfeed will not affect her future breast shape
one way or another. Heredity plays a large role in this matter, as
does excessive weight gain or loss.

Myth 2: Small-breasted women won't have enough milk.
Reality: The size of your breasts, either large or small, has nothing to
do with the amount of milk they will produce.

Myth 3: Today's artificial breast milk is just as good as the real thing.
Reality: Even though modern formulas are considerably better than
some of the old-fashioned ones, they can never replicate mother's
milk. In the first place, human milk contains live cells and human
hormones that are impossible to obtain from the mother's milk of

. . . by breathing deeply

Have you noticed something? Bet you aren't breathing. I don't mean
you aren't breathing at all – that, of course, would be impossible, but I
bet you hold your breath on a regular basis and 'forget' to breathe
properly. We all do it, apparently. The roots are in our caveman past.
When the tribe was in difficulty with a sabre-toothed tiger attack or a
wild marauding bunch of invading cavemen were on the prowl, we held
our breath to keep a low profile. Because rapid breath is part of the

another species. Research shows significant risk in the use of artificial milk.

Myth 4: Breastfeeding makes you fat.
Reality: Breastfeeding will certainly not prevent you from getting back to your pre-pregnancy weight. In fact, breastfeeding uses an extra 300–500 calories every day. It's up to the mother to choose how many of these calories she chooses to obtain through eating additional food or through burning off her available body fat. It is wise to lose weight gained during pregnancy gradually, whether or not you choose to breastfeed.

Myth 5: You can't get pregnant if you breastfeed.
Reality: True and false! Breastfeeding is only an effective form of birth control (98 per cent) during the first three months, and is only effective during this period if the baby is receiving nothing but breast milk on demand - no supplements, no solids, no water and no pacifiers. The chance of pregnancy increases greatly when a baby begins sleeping through the night, starts eating solids and/or when you resume your menstrual cycle. If you truly do not wish to become pregnant again yet, it is wise to use an additional method of birth control.

ancient flight or fight reaction, your body is preparing you for either fighting or fleeing.

Breathing is really important (now tell us something we don't know!) and although this should really be second nature for us by now, when we are under pressure it is one of the things that goes out the window. We rapidly shallow breathe in the top of our lungs, like little quivering voles, when we should be sucking in great big, generous, cat purring-like breaths of our life-giving nectar. This air gave your baby her first possibilities of life - what a miracle!

Now what did your mum tell you when you got your knickers in a twist when you were a wee nipper? She almost certainly said, 'Deep breath darling and count to three,' and she knew a thing your old mum, because breathing deeply is one certain way to calm down an over-wrought nervous system.

Actually, proper breathing is quite easy to do. It is just remembering to do it that is the problem.

* Take a deep breath in, imagining that you are filling a barrel with water, so that the barrel fills up from the bottom to the top. Your tummy should expand and you can feel the air fill your lungs right up to the top.
* Then breathe out through your nose.

Doesn't that feel great? Now get a sticky piece of paper, write on it 'BREATHE' and put in on the bathroom mirror. At least you will breathe every time you go for a pee. Try for a couple of really great breaths each time.

Here's another one to try and it's great for when junior is being more challenging than usual. It's called the anti-stress breath:

* Breathe in for 4 counts.
* Hold for 16 counts.
* Breathe out for 8 counts.

Feeling better? I thought so.

Be nice to yourself

* Get back your sanity and start breathing properly.
* Stick a really aesthetically ugly note on your bathroom mirror saying 'Breathe'.
* Don't hold your breath, it makes your face go red.

An expert speaks

Now obviously you might think that you do not have to actually learn how to breathe, since it is something we have done since birth. How wrong can we be? According to Kim Upton, an inspirational breath teacher, lots of us just don't know how to do it properly and are breathing all wrong, which can make us feel stressed out. To illustrate just what he means, Kim hooked me up to his magic machine that records how much carbon dioxide is in the system and in this way, he retrained me to breathe and therefore manage stress better. Before that I was holding my breath all the time – like some on strike kid who wants jelly and is not getting her own way. I didn't know that was what I was doing, but that was the effect.

The science of breathing is quite a lot more complex than we might imagine – taking in great big gulps of oxygen may seem like the right thing to do and, likewise, it seems logical to get rid of what's in the old lungs with the out puff (carbon dioxide mainly), but it turns out that we do need to retain some carbon dioxide to make good use of that all-important oxygen in our blood. And of course we need oxygen to live. This delicate balance is maintained or not, just by our breathing 'correctly'. Most of us, according to Kim, breathe in through our mouths and into only the upper part of the lungs, expanding the upper chest. As a result, we tend to rapidly over-breathe, making our body think that we are legging it at top speed from a particularly vicious woolly mammoth. When we breathe like this, stress levels rise and tension mounts and so daily life can seem like a constant emergency.

For you recently un-pregnant ladies, it may be interesting to learn that when you are nurturing that bump one of the main hormones whizzing around is progesterone, which is a breathing stimulant – all that rapid over-breathing can lower your carbon dioxide levels by up to 20 per cent so it's no wonder that a few of us go through the whole experience stressed out of our boxes. Not only that, but the growing baby increases the pressure on the diaphragm, which means you are even more likely to breathe from the upper chest. The problem is that after the birth you are still stuck in this stress-inducing loop, so it seems that you are already stressed before you actually are. Kim is passionate about teaching new mothers to break this cycle and to use proper breathing as one of the chief tools in the stress management armoury.

The trick is managing to keep carbon dioxide at the right level, which helps release tension in our muscles, which in turn then helps us to relax and digest food properly (*see* the top tips box, below).

Kim Upton's top tips for breathing right

❋ Practise breathing with the diaphragm by placing one hand on your upper chest and the other hand on your tummy. Lying down can help this.

❋ Visualise breathing in through the nose so that the breath reaches down to your hand resting on your abdomen and moving it out slightly.

❋ At the same time, allow your hand on your upper chest to relax and become still. Your hands act as guides to help 'feel' your breath. In time you will be able to do this naturally.

❋ Practise for ten minutes, twice a day, with a focus on relaxing the diaphragm and a gentle extension of your out breath. Avoid extending too far so as to 'grab' at the inhale and force yourself into upper chest breathing.

Of course, the right levels also say to our bodies that there isn't a woolly mammoth after us after all. Shame, I really, would love to see a woolly mammoth.

Win by a nose!

Kim tells me that your nose is your breathing's best friend. Breathing in through the nose or 'nose breathing', warms, moistens and filters the air for the lungs as well as regulating the amount of air you breath. You could say that the old adage 'less is more' is an underlying principle of good breathing and your nose is a good place to start.

You might feel that at first you are not getting enough air, but this will only take two or three days to change if you practise nose breathing regularly. Indeed, the aim is to nose breathe all the time. Persevere and you will find that it's the most natural way to breathe; as you were born to do so.

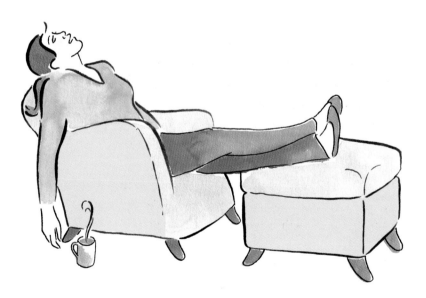

. . . by looking into after-pregnancy care with TCM

Naava Carman is quite simply a brilliant practitioner of Traditional Chinese Medicine (TCM). What is Traditional Chinese Medicine, I hear you cry? We in the West think we are awfully clever when it comes to medicine. Don't we know how to do heart surgery, bone marrow transplants, gender surgery, brain stuff? It is very, very clever and often saves countless lives, but in other societies they too have developed their own ways of keeping us healthy and in good shape and have been at it an awful lot longer than us – about 2,000–3,000 years longer in some cases. Many people are ready to dismiss what they don't know as hocus pocus, but even quite conservative circles are waking up to the benefits of alternative ways of making us well, or at the very least function better.

Traditional Chinese Medicine uses a mixture of herbal remedies and acupuncture (tiny needles placed on special points on the body to stimulate what they call qi – pronounced 'chi'). Qi is energy. I know you can't see energy and it is difficult sometimes for us doubting Thomases to believe in something we can't see, but lots of clever dudes over the millennia have worked this out. They also talk in different terms than our medical doctors. They might think that someone is damp or too hot or too cold, for example.

Naava specialises in fertility, so if you are even now thinking about having more kiddies (ha!), then Naava is the one to get you prepared and in good health. We often work together with good results – I do the nutrition and life bits and Naava does the TCM bits.

Restoring your periods with TCM

As a fertility and obstetric acupuncturist, Naava finds that one of the chief factors in helping a woman feel more 'herself' is the restoration of her periods, and this is helped along by something that is called 'mother roasting' in TCM. (I know that doesn't sound tempting folks, but it is just an expression so don't panic. You will not be trussed up, basted and made into a main course.)

Mother roasting is done by using a herb called moxa or mugwort, which is tightly packed into a stick. If you can persuade your partner to come along to an appointment with your TCM practitioner, so much the better as the acupuncturist will demonstrate how to light the stick and move it in a figure-of-eight over the mother's lower belly. It looks a bit like a cigar. Doing this daily from about three weeks after the birth helps to contract the uterus to its optimum level, as well as helping stop any bleeding after the birth and can help shape up the uterus.

Overcoming mastitis with TCM

Naava finds that mastitis is also a common issue that women suffer from during the initial phases of breastfeeding. She finds that often the Staphylococcus aureus infection is passed from baby to mother (from the baby's mouth) and back again, and this can often lead to a vicious cycle, which means that mothers have pain with breastfeeding, lumps in the milk ducts and even fever and infection themselves. The conventional method is to give antibiotics and continue to breastfeed, which helps to drain away the infection. This works well in some mothers, while others find that the antibiotics can cause other side effects, such as thrush in themselves, constipation or diarrhoea in the baby and, in some cases, have no lasting effect.

There are certain herbs that can break the cycle of infection and, providing the herbalist is properly qualified and a member of the Register of Chinese Herbal Medicine (RCHM), then the herbs will be safe to use while breastfeeding and will all be baby friendly. Practitioners work on the principle that the imbalance in the mother that necessitates the herbs will be affecting the child, too. Conversely, by giving herbs that redress the imbalance, the child's health will also be positively affected.

TCM practitioner Naava's top tips for mastitis

* Keep breastfeeding. Although this may be uncomfortable initially, it will help in the long term to keep the flow of milk available and clear the heat from infection.

* Use a wheat-pack. These are available in many health food stores and can be heated in the microwave for expediency. A few minutes before and during a feed, place the pack on the affected breast and, if necessary, over the lump in the breast and keep it there until feeding is finished. This will give topical relief.

* Massage the breast and lymph nodes under the arm to help move the blocked qi (energy) in the ducts.

* Find a Chinese herbalist through the Register of Chinese Herbal Medicine (www.rchm.co.uk). All herbalists who are members have gone through a level of training that will include pharmacology and will be obtaining their herbs through an RCHM recommended source. A herbalist should be able to make a difference to mastitis within 24–48 hours.

Helping 'the blues' with TCM

In Naava's experience, depression is something many women experience in varying forms. This might take the form of profound fatigue and complete loss of libido, even after the baby gets into a routine that lets you sleep, or it might be something as small as a tendency to weepiness and feeling easily unsettled emotionally. The best way to find an acupuncturist who can deal with depression after birth is through the British Acupuncture Council (BAcC). Visit www.acupuncture.org.uk.

Acupressure points

Here are some acupressure points you can use at home to help you feel less blue.

* There is a very powerful pressure point on the wrists that has a calming effect on the mind and is also excellent for depression that is accompanied by a feeling of anxiety in the pit of the stomach. Rather than try to find the point yourself, you can buy a travel sickness band and wear it, as it will stimulate the correct point and provide some relief for you.

* Rub around your navel in a clockwise direction – this acts as a calming and grounding action. For some women, this will precipitate a cathartic bout of crying but don't fear, you will feel much better afterwards!

* Make sure your lower back is warm – this is the kidney area in TCM and the kidneys are responsible for making sure that your foundation of qi (energy) is strong. The kidney energy is also responsible for conception, so after you have given birth, they are a bit depleted and can use all the help they can get. If the area is warm, it is a good sign that they are looking after themselves well.

Be nice to yourself

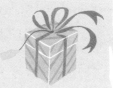

* Try something new. Why not try TCM or some other alternative therapy? Again, recommendations are the best way to find a good practitioner.

* If you are feeling low, get a good movie out and laugh – it's so easy to lose perspective. Let your mind drift elsewhere for a few hours

* If you are feeling really low, ask for help. Don't stew in your own juice.

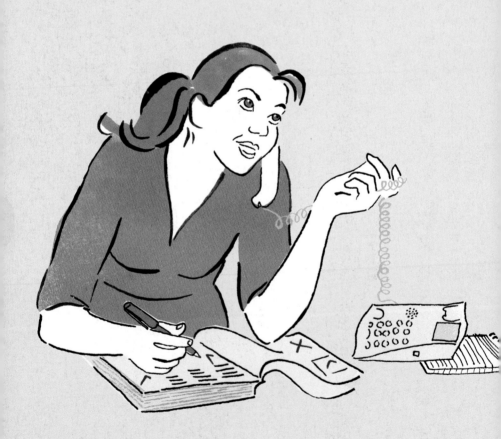

The final bit

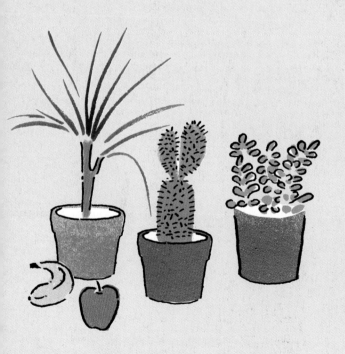

The final bit

You can do it. Remember, if you have other problems address them, but eating can become a pleasure and not a battle ground. You can reach your goals, even without too much effort. Here's Lisa's story.

Lisa's story

After having my gorgeous boy, Blake, and 18 months down the line I really thought it was time to get both my body and sanity back. Nobody tells you how tiring it is looking after an energetic toddler, working and looking after a home. I was exhausted and had never really got back to my pre-birth weight either. Also, as a sufferer of IBS for over ten years I was beginning to despair. My symptoms started in my twenties and took me completely by surprise. I was quite ill and would suffer from fatigue and severe stomach cramps that required hospitalization, as well as the more common symptoms. Until I was properly diagnosed, I was given many variables on what the problem could be. I had seen several specialists but the advice was always to maintain such a severe diet that it was impossible to live a normal life. I wanted to hang out with my friends, but this was getting in the way. I tried to ignore it, but the symptoms would not go away and they were getting worse. I was resigned to living on rice cakes and tahini! After becoming pregnant and suffering nine months of severe stomach discomfort I decided to take the matter in hand once I gave birth. I was not getting any younger and wanted to be healthy for me and my new family.

I met Kate some years before I finally booked a consultation. At the time I was wary of booking an appointment because I thought that she would be unable to help and I would be back to eating rice cakes morning, noon and night. As luck would have it, Kate joined our team of practitioners when I returned from my maternity leave. I thought it must be fate and decided to put all my reservations aside and tell her what was going on with me.

I have to say it was the best thing I could have done, she was truly fantastic. She listened and did not make me feel bad about my poor eating habits. My biggest fear was being told I would have to live on a ridiculous diet for the rest of my life but what she said was so sensible and logical. We went through my whole history and eating habits. She gave me one task and that was to eat breakfast. Simple you think, but something I never did on a regular basis. I could eat what I wanted but I had advice on alternatives that would help alleviate my IBS symptoms.

It has worked amazingly; I can honestly say Kate changed my way of thinking about food completely. Not only do I feel heaps better, but I also lost over 18 pounds without having to spend ten hours a week at the gym – something I had been trying to do since giving birth to my son. I feel great and have a lot more energy as a working mum. My biggest achievement is that I do not crave chocolate anymore, something that I was addicted to and thought I could never give up. I don't stress about food and for the first time I am really happy about my eating habits. I have applied some of this new eating ethic to my whole family and it is making a big difference. My son sleeps much better, which is a big help to me. If Kate can recommend a food source that stops my husband snoring, I would be eternally grateful!

Thanks Kate, I am a changed woman because of you. As Kate says to me, 'Go well' and that's exactly what I intend to keep on doing.

Good luck to everyone and please, good health and ...

... go well!

Kate

Resources

Shopping list

* Choose organic when possible, especially grains, meat, dairy and root vegetables. Remember, food that is the most fragile or has to look the most presentable, e.g. strawberries, lettuce, will be the most heavily sprayed.
* Choose foods in season where possible and include a variety of colours (include traffic-light colours on your plate) and experiment with new foods for a range of nutrients. Use raw vegetables where possible as they are rich in enzymes that can aid digestion.
* Shop online at Waitrose, Sainsbury, Tesco and Asda.

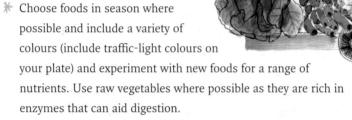

Grains: Brown basmati rice, buckwheat, millet, quinoa, barley.

Pastas: Buckwheat, kamut, millet, rice and corn. Spelt & Hemp pasta by Mother Hemp is a delicious alternative.

Nuts: Almonds, Brazils, cashews, hazelnuts, pecans, pinenuts and walnuts.

Seeds: Hemp, linseeds, pumpkin, sesame and sunflower.

Breads & crackers: Rye, spelt, rice bread, Stamp Collection breads (wheat free), Ryvita, oatcakes, rice cakes, corn cakes, Village Bakery Savoury Biscuits (gluten free).

Seasonings: Fresh and dried herbs, sea salt, pepper, tamari, olives, pesto (check labels, many contain cheese), Braggs liquid aminos (soya sauce alternative), cider vinegar, lemon, lime, chilli, ginger, spices, onions and garlic. Cinnamon and nutmeg for porridge and fruit dishes.

Oils: Extra virgin olive oil, flaxseed*, hemp seed* and pumpkin seed oil*, sesame, walnut and unrefined sunflower oil. (*don't use to cook with, add to food after cooking).

Cupboard basics: Lentils, chickpeas, butterbeans, tinned tomatoes, sweetcorn, artichokes, sundried tomatoes and tuna. Soya, nut, rice (Rice Dream) and oat (Oatly) milk. Whole grain cereal, no-added sugar muesli and porridge oats.

Flours & baking products: Ground chestnut flour, wholemeal wheatflour, baked beans (check labels for sugar and salt content), soya, rye, tapioca, rice, potato, quinoa, gram, buckwheat, ground cornmeal and spelt. Baking powder (use xanthan gum if you're avoiding gluten).

Freezer basics: Vegetables; peas, spinach, sweetcorn, cauliflower, broad beans, Brussels sprouts and green beans. Mixed berries, raspberries, blueberries and cranberries. Chicken, turkey and fish.

Fridge Basics: Fresh vegetables, live yoghurt (Provamel soya if you're avoiding dairy), nut butters, smoothies (Innocent have a good range), organic free-range eggs, fresh fish and organic unsalted butter.

Enjoy!

A few great sites for online food shopping

www.abel-cole.co.uk
Organic home delivery boxes. Nationwide delivery, check availability by typing in your postcode.

www.alotoforganics.co.uk
UK organic search engine.

www.asda.com
Deliveries in two-hour slots. 10am–10pm Monday to Saturday and 11am–8pm on Sundays.

www.bercoeli.com
Gluten- and wheat-free products.

www.bigbarn.co.uk
A comprehensive list of shops and markets in your area (type in your postcode).

www.crayves.co.uk
Organic and special dietary needs breads, cakes and crackers.

www.foodferry.com
Food and grocery shopping delivered to your door; London only.

www.goodnessdirect.co.uk
A wide range of foods including special dietary needs, beverages, toiletries and households products.

www.ocado.com (Waitrose)
Deliveries within a one hour delivery slot. 7am–10pm, six days a week.

www.organicdelivery.co.uk
Organic foods and a range of household goods; delivered in the London area.

www.organicfood.co.uk
Local sources for organic produce.

www.orgran.com
Offers information, mail order and recipes.

www.realproduce.co.uk
Information on farmers markets, places to eat, books, recipes and a 'where to shop' guide.

www.sainsburys.com
Deliveries in two-hour slots. 7am–10pm, seven days a week.

www.tesco.com
Deliveries in two-hour slots. 9am–11pm Monday to Saturday and 10am–3pm on Sundays.

www.vegansociety.com
Their official website.

www.vegsoc.org (Vegetarian Society)
Cookery courses and schools, recipes, food facts and advice on eating out.

www.village-bakery.com
A comprehensive range of wheat-free, gluten-free and dairy-free breads, crackers and more.

www.zedzfoods.co.uk
Offers information, mail order and recipes

Other recommended sites

www.parkfarmorganics.co.uk
www.graigfarm.co.uk
www.localfoodweb.co.uk
www.farmersmarkets.net Provides a comprehensive list of markets in your area.

Education and advice

www.laleche.org.uk
For friendly mother-to-mother breastfeeding support from pregnancy through to weaning.

www.nct.org.uk
National Childbirth Trust is the leading charity dealing with pregnancy, birth and early parenthood in the UK, operating at both local and national levels across Scotland, England, Wales and Northern Ireland.

www.parentlineplus.org.uk
Parentline Plus works to offer help and support through an innovative range of free, flexible, responsive services – shaped by parents for parents – because children don't come with instructions!

Healthy living

www.ecobaby.co.uk
Home of shopping for natural skincare products for baby, child and you. They are a small family run site dedicated to bringing caring parents a great choice of products.

www.healthyhouse.co.uk
Suppliers of allergy-free clothing, bedding and other household items.

www.soilassociation.org
The UK's leading environmental charity promoting sustainable, organic farming and championing human health. They provide a directory of where to buy organic food, from farm shops and box-delivery schemes to organic retailers.

Nutritional care

www.biocare.co.uk
A wide range of vitamins and minerals for breastfeeding mothers, babies and children.

www.healthplus.co.uk
Supplements designed for pre, during and post pregnancy.

www.thenutritioncoach.co.uk
The Nutrition Coach is born out of the practical knowledge that although we may have a sincere wish to change our eating plans, the reality is often difficult to achieve without on-going support. With the support of a qualified nutritionist, The Nutrition Coach makes it easier to take your health into your own hands.

www.vitacare.co.uk
Goat-milk based nutritional products, including NannyCare Infant Milk formula.

Services

www.buetykohealth.com
Kim Upton MBIBH, is a breathing rehabilitation specialist and buteyko practitioner

www.davidsamson.co.uk
David Samson, Dip. Adv. Hyp., is a clinical hypnotherapist specialising in hypnosis for weight loss, stop smoking, depression, insomnia, IBS, fear of flying, self-confidence, panic attacks and phobias.

www.fertilitysupportcompany.co.uk
Navaa Carman provides comprehensive healthcare for men and women wishing to become parents.

www.lucywyndhamread.com
Lucy is a personal fitness consultant specialising in designing workouts you can do from your home. She is qualified in pre- and post-natal exercise instruction.

www.thebirthcompany.co.uk
The Birth Company is a leading London women's pregnancy and childbirth clinic, specialising in obstetrics from single scans to full specialist pregnancy care and general gynaecology care.

Index